CHAIR YOGA

FOR SENIORS OVER 60

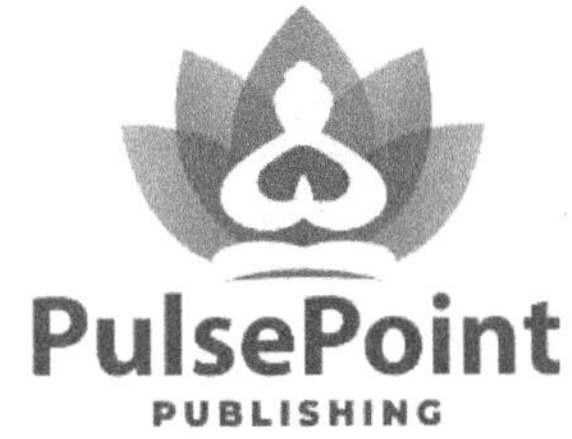

PulsePoint
PUBLISHING

GET YOUR
EXTRA CONTENT
NOW!

To download the digital version of these bonuses you don't need to enter any details except your name and email address.

EXTRA#1
+170 VIDEO TUTORIALS

EXTRA#2
5 PLANNERS & JOURNALS

Simply scan the QR code below
or go to

bonusbookshelf.com/pulsepoint-publishing-cy

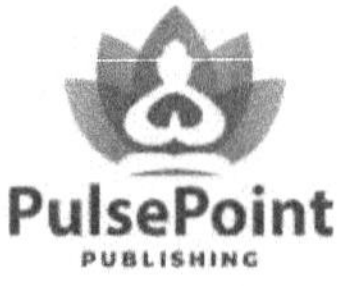

Table of Contents

CHAPTER 1: INTRODUCTION TO CHAIR YOGA

Chair yoga is a specialized form of yoga that has been specifically designed for seniors, offering a gentle and accessible way to experience the benefits of yoga. This practice involves performing various yoga poses and exercises while seated on a chair, making it suitable for individuals with limited mobility or physical limitations.

1. Benefits of Chair Yoga for Seniors

Chair yoga provides numerous benefits for seniors, enhancing their overall well-being and quality of life. One of the key advantages of this is its ability to improve flexibility, strength, and balance. Through a series of gentle movements and stretches, chair yoga helps to increase the range of motion in joints, making daily activities easier and reducing the risk of injury.

Moreover, chair yoga is an effective way to build strength in the muscles, particularly in the core, arms, and legs. By engaging in regular practice, seniors can strengthen their muscles, which in turn helps to support their posture and stability.

In addition to flexibility and strength, chair yoga also promotes better balance. As we age, maintaining balance becomes increasingly important to prevent falls and injuries. Chair yoga incorporates specific exercises that target balance, such as seated leg lifts and side stretches, helping seniors to improve their stability and reduce the risk of falls.

2. Techniques and Modifications of Chair Yoga Poses

Chair yoga modifies traditional yoga poses to make them accessible and safe for seniors. The use of a chair provides support and stability, allowing individuals to comfortably perform the poses without putting strain on their joints or muscles.

Some common chair yoga poses include:

• Seated Mountain Pose: Sit up tall in the chair, grounding your feet on the floor. Place your hands on your thighs and focus on stretching your spine and relaxing your shoulders.

• Seated Forward Bend: Sit on the edge of the chair, feet hip-width apart. Slowly bend forward from your hips, bringing your hands to your feet on the floor. This position stretches both the hamstrings and the lower back.

• Seated Twist: Sit sideways on the chair, with one hand holding onto the backrest. Gently twist your torso towards the backrest, keeping your spine long and your core engaged. Repeat on the other side.

These are just a few examples of the many chair yoga poses that can be incorporated into a senior's daily routine. The modifications allow individuals to experience the benefits of yoga while adapting to their physical capabilities and limitations.

3. Reducing Stress and Promoting Relaxation

Chair yoga not only improves physical well-being but also has a positive impact on mental and emotional health. Engaging in this kind of exercise can help seniors reduce stress, anxiety, and tension by focusing on deep breathing and mindful movements.

The slow and controlled nature of chair yoga allows individuals to connect with their breath and bring a sense of calmness into their daily lives. By incorporating relaxation techniques into the practice, such as guided meditation or visualization, chair yoga provides a holistic approach to stress reduction and promotes a greater sense of relaxation and well-being.

4. Making Yoga Accessible to All

One of the most significant advantages of chair yoga is its ability to make yoga accessible to individuals with limited mobility or physical limitations. By utilizing a chair, individuals who may have difficulty getting up and down from the floor can still participate in the practice and enjoy its benefits.

Chair yoga may be done in a variety of locations, including community centers, senior centers, and even at home. It offers a safe and inclusive environment for seniors to engage in physical activity, improve their overall health, and connect with others in their community.

The Concept, History, and Benefits of Chair Yoga for Seniors.

Chair yoga for seniors is a wonderful practice that combines the benefits of yoga with the comfort and support of a chair. It is a gentle form of exercise that can be easily incorporated into daily life, making it accessible to seniors of all fitness levels.

Chair yoga has its roots in traditional yoga, which originated in ancient India thousands of years ago. Over time, yoga has evolved and adapted to meet the needs of different individuals, including seniors who may have limited mobility or balance. Chair yoga provides a safe and effective way for seniors to experience the physical and mental benefits of yoga without the need to get down on the floor.

The benefits of chair yoga for seniors are numerous and wide-ranging. First and foremost, it promotes flexibility and strength. Chair yoga involves moderate motions and stretches that promote joint mobility and muscle tone. This is particularly important for seniors, as maintaining flexibility and strength can help prevent falls and injuries.

Chair yoga encourages relaxation and stress reduction. Slow and controlled motions, paired with concentrated breathing methods, assist to relax the mind and body. This is especially helpful for seniors who may be anxious or have difficulties sleeping.

In addition to physical and mental benefits, chair yoga also offers social and emotional benefits. Participating in a chair yoga session allows seniors to interact with others and foster a feeling of community. It can also boost self-esteem and confidence, as individuals see improvements in their physical abilities and overall well-being.

Before beginning a chair yoga practice, elders should visit their healthcare physician. They can give advice on any unique concerns or measures that must be addressed based on individual health issues or limits. It is also critical to select a trained instructor who has prior experience dealing with elders and can make necessary changes and adaptations.

While this guide provides a comprehensive overview of chair yoga for seniors, it does not provide specific information on different poses and techniques used in chair yoga. However, there are numerous resources available, including books, videos, and online classes, that can provide detailed instructions and demonstrations of chair yoga poses.

For seniors, chair yoga is a beneficial practice that offers a gentle and accessible way to experience the physical and mental benefits of yoga. It is important for seniors to consult with their healthcare provider before starting a chair yoga practice and to find a qualified instructor who can provide guidance and modifications. By incorporating chair yoga into their daily lives, seniors can improve flexibility, strength, and overall well-being, while also enjoying the social and emotional benefits of this wonderful practice.

CHAPTER 2: CHAIR YOGA AND THE AGING PROCESS

One of the key advantages of chair yoga is its accessibility. Unlike traditional yoga, which often involves standing or lying on the floor, chair yoga allows individuals with limited mobility or balance issues to participate fully. The use of a chair provides stability and support, making it easier for older adults to perform the various poses and exercises.

Regular chair yoga practice has been shown to alleviate common age-related issues such as joint pain, stiffness, and reduced mobility. The gentle movements and stretches involved in chair yoga help to increase joint flexibility and range of motion. This can lead to a reduction in discomfort and an improvement in overall joint health.

In addition to physical benefits, chair yoga has a good impact on mental health. The practice includes deep breathing and mindfulness practices, which can help decrease tension and promote relaxation. This can be particularly beneficial for older adults who may be experiencing increased levels of stress or anxiety.

When practicing chair yoga, there are a variety of poses and exercises that can be performed. These include seated twists, forward bends, side stretches, and gentle backbends. Each pose is designed to target specific areas of the body and promote strength, flexibility, and balance.

Physical Benefits of Chair Yoga

Chair yoga offers numerous physical benefits for older adults. This modified form of yoga is designed to be practiced while seated, making it accessible for individuals with limited mobility or balance issues. Regular practice of chair yoga can lead to significant improvements in flexibility, strength, balance, and overall well-being in older adults.

One of the primary physical benefits of chair yoga is increased flexibility. The gentle stretching exercises performed in chair yoga help to increase the range of motion in the joints, making everyday movements easier and more comfortable. By doing chair yoga, seniors can experience reduced joint pain and stiffness, allowing them to move more freely and engage in daily activities with greater ease.

Chair yoga also helps to enhance strength in older adults. The various poses and movements target different muscle groups, helping to build strength and stability. Strong muscles are necessary for keeping appropriate posture and avoiding falls, which are typical concerns among seniors. Chair yoga helps elderly persons develop their muscles and increase their overall physical power.

Another physical benefit is improved balance. Many chair yoga poses focus on stability and core strength, which are essential for maintaining balance and preventing falls. By practicing these poses regularly, older adults can improve their balance and reduce the risk of accidents and injuries. Enhanced balance Not only does it promote physical well-being, but it also increases confidence and independence in everyday tasks.

Regular chair yoga practice also has positive effects on joint health. The gentle movements and stretches in chair yoga help to lubricate the joints and increase blood flow, promoting joint health and reducing the risk of age-related conditions such as arthritis. Seniors who practice chair yoga may experience reduced joint pain and increased mobility, allowing them to engage in activities they enjoy with greater comfort.

In addition to the physical benefits, chair yoga improves mental health in older persons. Chair yoga classes emphasize deep breathing and mindfulness, which assist to relieve tension and promote relaxation. This can have a good effect on general mental health by lowering anxiety and enhancing mood. Chair yoga is a relaxing and refreshing practice that helps elders achieve peace and quiet.

To reap the physical benefits of chair yoga, it is recommended to practice two to three times per week for 20 to 30 minutes each session. Consistency is key to experience the positive effects on flexibility, strength, balance, and overall well-being. Chair yoga is a valuable tool for promoting healthy aging and improving physical health in older adults.

Emotional Well-being and Yoga

Chair yoga not only has physical benefits for seniors but also plays a significant role in improving their emotional well-being. Seniors often face emotional challenges such as stress, anxiety, and mood swings, and practicing chair yoga can help them cope with these challenges effectively.

One of the key ways chair yoga promotes emotional well-being in seniors is through stress reduction. The gentle stretching and breathing exercises involved in chair yoga help activate the body's relaxation response, which can counteract the effects of stress. By focusing on the present moment and engaging in slow, controlled movements, seniors can experience a sense of calm and relaxation. This can lead to a reduction in stress levels and an overall improvement in emotional well-being.

Chair yoga also enhances mood and promotes a positive mindset. The combination of physical movement, deep breathing, and mindfulness can stimulate the release of endorphins, which are natural mood-boosting chemicals in the brain. Regular practice of chair yoga can help seniors experience more positive emotions, reduce feelings of sadness or depression, and improve their overall outlook on life.

In addition to stress reduction and mood enhancement, chair yoga can contribute to overall mental health in seniors. The practice encourages mindfulness and self-awareness, allowing seniors to connect with their emotions and thoughts in a non-judgmental way. This increased self-awareness can help seniors better understand and manage their emotional challenges. Chair yoga provides a safe and supportive environment for seniors to explore their emotions and develop strategies for emotional well-being.

Specific chair yoga poses and techniques can be particularly beneficial for seniors in managing their emotional challenges. Poses such as the seated forward bend, gentle twists, and chest openers can help release tension and promote relaxation. Deep breathing exercises, such as the three-part breath or alternate nostril breathing, can help seniors regulate their emotions and find inner calm. Mindfulness techniques, such as body scans or guided imagery, can also be incorporated into chair yoga sessions to promote emotional well-being.

Overall, chair yoga is not only a physical practice but also a powerful tool for improving emotional well-being in seniors. By reducing stress, enhancing mood, and promoting overall mental health, chair yoga can help seniors effectively cope with emotional challenges. The specific poses and techniques used in chair yoga provide seniors with the means to manage their emotions and cultivate a positive mindset.

To reap the physical and emotional benefits of chair yoga, it is recommended for seniors to practice regularly; ideally two to three times per week for 20–30 minutes each session. Consistency is key to experiencing the positive effects on flexibility, strength, balance, emotional and overall well-being. Chair yoga is a valuable tool for promoting healthy aging and improving physical health in older adults and can lead to improved emotional well-being and a greater sense of overall happiness and contentment.

CHAPTER 3: INTEGRATING CHAIR YOGA INTO DAILY LIFE

There are other benefits associated with chair yoga, including improved flexibility, reduces stress levels and overall well-being. Even though it is performed seated, there are variations of each exercise and modifications can be made to accommodate different levels of fitness, allowing individuals to customize their chair yoga practice bases on their abilities.

Integrating chair yoga into various daily activities is encouraged. It can be done whether at a desk, during work breaks, while watching TV or even while engaging in other leisure activities.

Setting Up for Chair Yoga

Creating a safe and effective home space for chair yoga is essential to ensure a comfortable and beneficial practice. Here are some practical tips and advice to help you set up your space:

1. Find a suitable chair: Choose a sturdy chair without wheels that provides good support for your back. Avoid chairs with armrests that are too high or wide, as they may restrict movement during certain poses.

2. Clear the area: Make sure you have enough space around the chair to move freely without any obstructions. Remove any objects or furniture that may interfere with your practice.

3. Use a non-slip mat: Place a non-slip yoga mat or rug under the chair to prevent it from sliding during your practice. This will improve stability and lower the danger of accidents.

4. Adjust the height: If necessary, adjust the height of the chair to ensure that your feet are flat on the ground and your knees are at a 90-degree angle. This will assist keep your joints in optimal alignment and reduce strain.

5. Create a calming atmosphere: Dim the lights or use soft lighting to create the desired atmosphere. Play soothing music or nature sounds to create a tranquil environment that promotes relaxation and attention.

6. Gather props: Depending on your comfort and flexibility level, you may want to have additional props nearby. This can include yoga blocks, blankets, or straps to assist with certain poses or modifications.

7. Dress comfortably: Wear loose, airy clothes that allows for free mobility. Avoid wearing any jewelry or accessories that might interfere with your practice.

8. Warm up and cool down: Begin your chair yoga practice with a gentle warm-up to prepare your body for movement. Similarly, end your practice with a cooling-down period to relax and restore your body.

9. Practice mindfulness: Before starting your chair yoga session, take a few moments to center yourself and focus on your breath. Stay in the present moment and let go of any distractions or worry.

10. Stay hydrated: Keep a bottle of water nearby to remain hydrated during your practice. It is critical to restore fluids and sustain proper bodily function.

By following these guidelines, you can create a safe and inviting space for your chair yoga practice. Remember to listen to your body, respect your limits, and enjoy the numerous physical and mental benefits that chair yoga has to offer.

Personalizing Yoga Practices

Understanding the unique needs and abilities of individuals is crucial when it comes to practicing yoga. Tailoring chair yoga routines to suit different body types, modifying poses for specific conditions or injuries, and customizing the intensity and duration of the practice are all important components to consider when creating a routine.

To begin personalizing yoga practices, it is important to have a clear understanding of different body types. Each body type has its own strengths, limitations, and areas of focus. By recognizing these differences, individuals can modify poses and sequences to ensure a safe and effective practice. For example, individuals with a larger body type may need to use props or modify poses to accommodate their size, while those with a smaller body type may need to focus on building strength and stability.

In addition to body types, it is also necessary to consider any specific conditions or injuries that individuals may have. Yoga can be adapted to accommodate various conditions such as arthritis, back pain, or joint injuries. By modifying poses and using props, individuals can still experience the benefits of yoga while working within their limitations. It is important to consult with a healthcare professional or a qualified yoga instructor to ensure that the modifications are appropriate and safe.

Another aspect of personalizing chair yoga practices is customizing the intensity and duration of the practice. Some individuals may require a more gentle and restorative practice, while others may prefer a more vigorous and challenging routine. By adjusting the pace, duration, and difficulty level of the poses, individuals can create a practice that suits their energy levels and goals. It is important to listen to the body and make modifications as needed to avoid overexertion or strain.

To help individuals personalize their chair yoga practices, here are some key considerations to keep in mind:

1. Focus on individual body type and modify poses accordingly.

2. Use props such as blocks, bolsters, or blankets to support and enhance the practice.

3. Pay attention to any specific conditions or injuries and modify poses to accommodate them.

4. Customize the intensity and duration of the practice based on energy levels and goals.

5. Practice mindfulness and listen to the body's signals to avoid overexertion.

6. Seek guidance from a qualified yoga instructor or healthcare professional for personalized modifications.

To provide a practical example, here is a personalized chair yoga routine for an individual with arthritis:

7. Begin with gentle neck stretches, moving the head from side to side and up and down.

8. Proceed to shoulder rolls, moving the shoulders forward and backward to relieve tension.

9. Perform seated spinal twists, gently twisting the upper body from side to side.

10. Practice seated forward bends, reaching forward to stretch the hamstrings and lower back.

11. Incorporate wrist and ankle rotations to improve joint mobility.

12. Finish with a guided relaxation, focusing on deep breathing and releasing tension in the body.

Individuals may adjust their chair yoga practices to their own requirements and goals by customizing them. This makes the yoga experience more joyful and useful, boosting both physical and emotional well-being.

Stretch

1 - Low Lunge Backbend

Goal: Stretch the lats and the chest

Difficulty: ★★★☆☆

Description: A gentle lunge pose with one both legs bent, incorporating a backward stretch with hands interlaced behind the back.

Step-by-step:

1. Begin with one thigh resting on the chair, and the foot planted on the floor. The opposite leg is in front of the chair at 90 degrees.

2. Engage your core.

3. Keep your front knee directly over your ankle and your back toes tucked under, ensuring stability and alignment.

4. Interlace your hands behind your back or grab opposite elbows. Inhale as you pull your hands back, lifting your chest and allowing your gaze to follow.

5. Stay in this backbend and continue to breathe.

6. Ensure your hips remain squared and your tailbone lengthens down toward the chair to protect your lower back.

7. Hold the pose for 30–45 seconds.

8. Repeat on the opposite side, swapping leg positions.

9. After completing both sides, return to a seated position and take a moment to notice any sensations in your body.

10. Repeat 3–5 times.

Scan the QR code below for the video tutorial

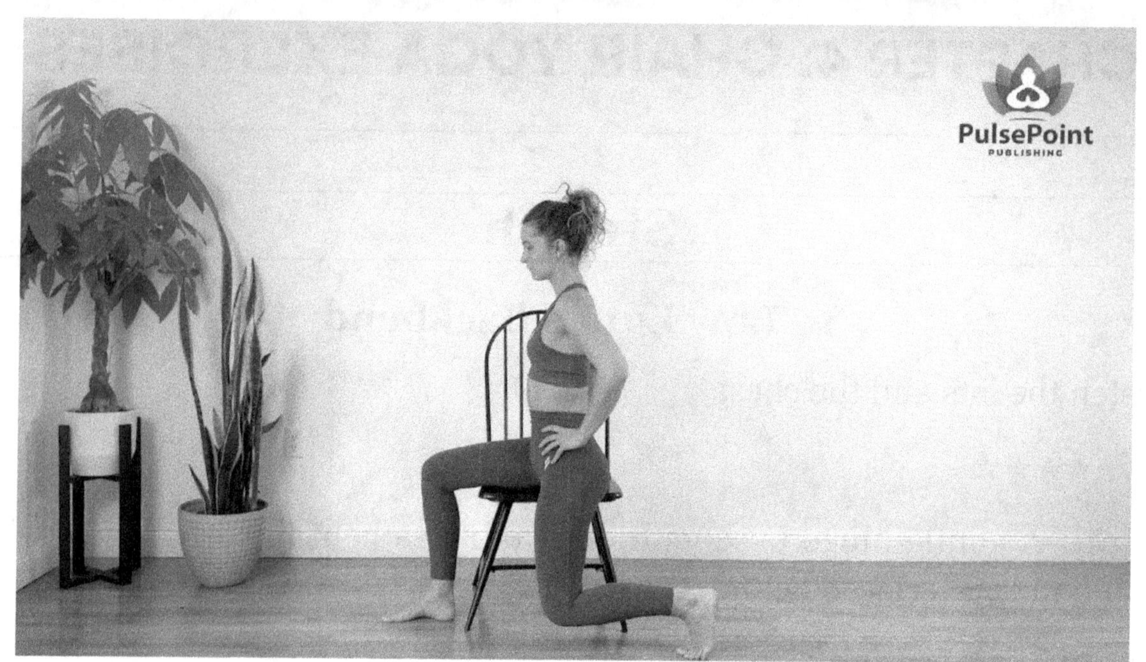

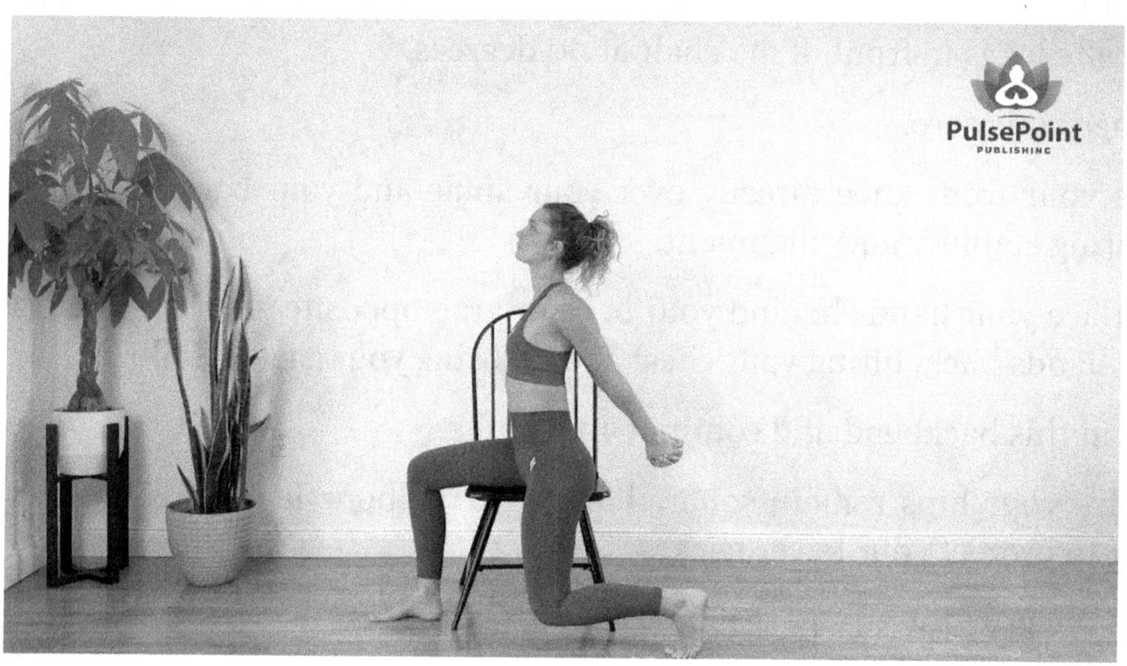

2 - Half Split

Goal: Stretch the hamstrings

Difficulty: ★★★★☆

Description: A standing stretch where one leg is extended, emphasizing a deep stretch for the hamstring by leaning forward over the extended leg.

Step-by-step:

1. Begin standing behind your chair with your feet hip-width apart, facing forward and holding onto the back of the chair for support.

2. Use core muscles to support your body.

3. Lift one foot onto the chair and extend it straight, resting the heel.

4. Flex your lifted foot and keep your hips squared towards the chair to ensure proper alignment.

5. Inhale, lengthen the spine, stand tall.

6. Exhale, hinge forward at your hips, folding over the extended leg while maintaining a straight spine.

7. Continue to hold onto the chair for support or challenge your balance by extending your arms straight out in front of you or placing your hands on your hips.

8. Hold for 30–45 seconds, focusing on maintaining balance and lengthening through the back of your grounded leg.

9. Repeat 3–5 times.

Scan the QR code below for the video tutorial

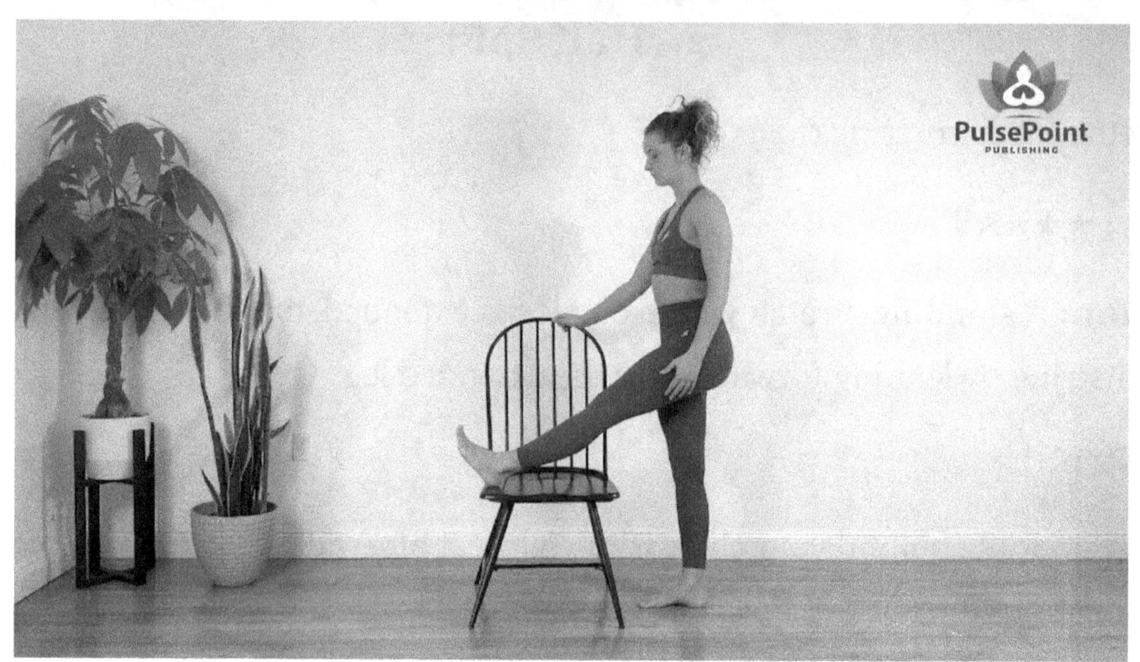

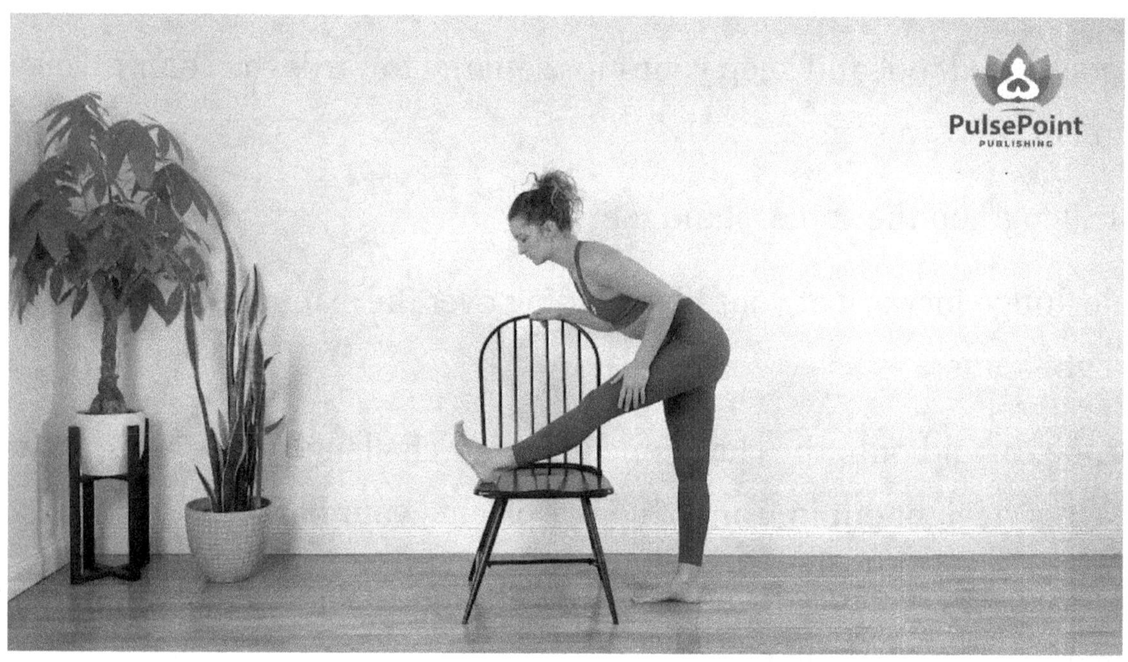

3 - Seated Forward Fold

Goal: Stretch the hips and low back

Difficulty: ★★☆☆☆

Description: A seated position where the upper body folds forward from the hips, targeting the back and hips for flexibility and relaxation.

Step-by-step:

1. Begin seated at the front edge of your chair with your feet flat on the floor, hip-width apart.
2. Sit up tall, lengthening your spine, and place your hands on your thighs for support.
3. Take a deep inhale, lifting your arms overhead, reaching towards the ceiling.
4. Exhale as you slowly hinge forward at your hips, leading with your chest, and lowering your torso towards your thighs.
5. Rest your hands on your shins, ankles, or the floor based on your flexibility.
6. Keep your spine long and your shoulders relaxed away from your ears.
7. Let your head hang heavy, releasing any tension in your neck.
8. Take slow, deep breaths as you hold the pose, allowing gravity to gently deepen the stretch.
9. Relax into the forward fold, surrendering to the sensation of the stretch in your hamstrings and lower back.
10. Hold the pose for 30 seconds, breathing deeply and consciously.
11. To release, engage your core muscles and slowly roll up through your spine, stacking each vertebra one at a time until you are sitting upright.
12. Repeated 3–5 times.

Scan the QR code below for the video tutorial

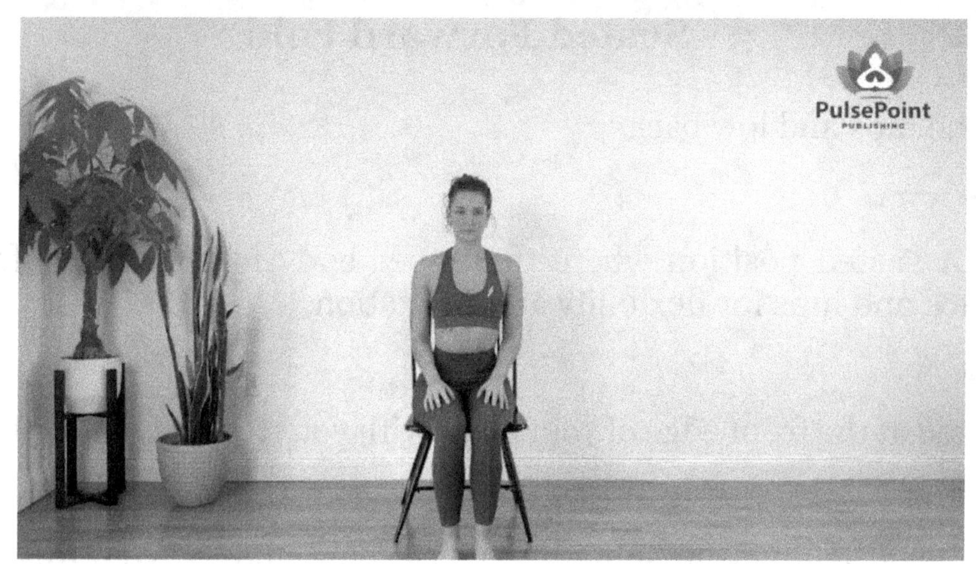

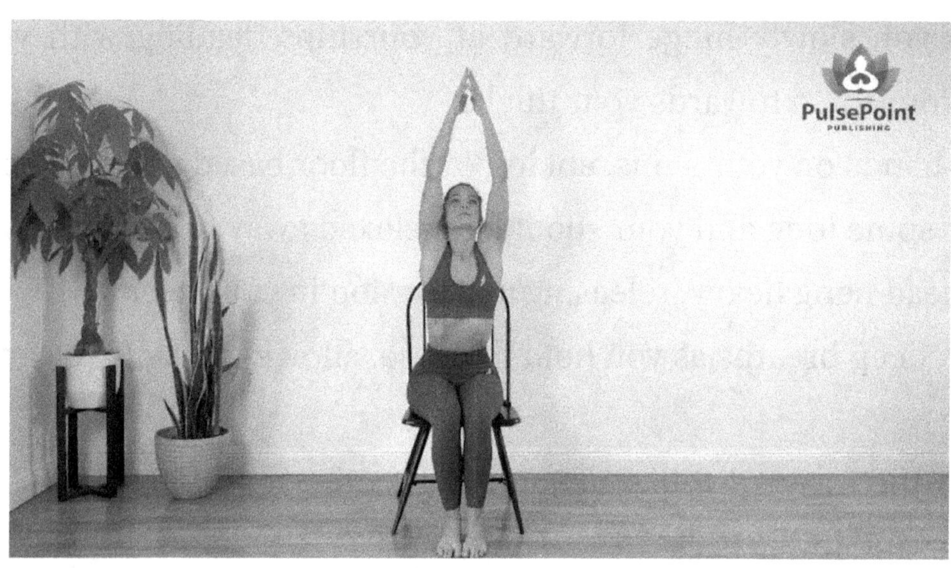

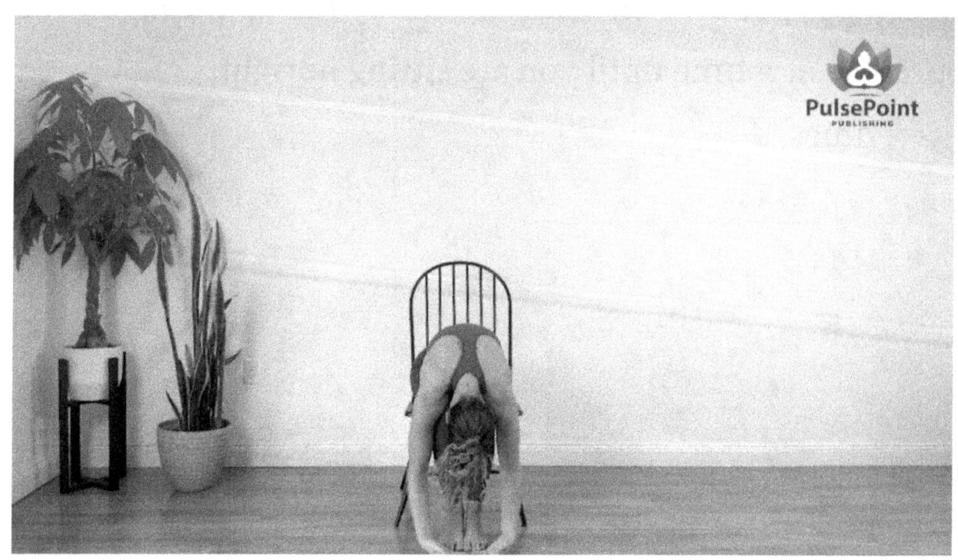

4 - Seated Pigeon

Goal: Stretch the hips and glutes

Difficulty: ★★★★☆

Description: A modified seated stretch, where one ankle is crossed over the opposite thigh.

Step-by-step:

1. Begin seated on the edge of your chair with your feet flat on the floor, hip-width apart.
2. Sit up tall, lengthening your spine, and place your hands on your thighs for support.
3. Lift one foot off the floor and cross your right ankle over your opposite knee, allowing your right knee to open out to the side.
4. Flex your crossed foot to protect your knee and engage your muscles.
5. Stay in this position to feel a gentle stretch in your right outer hip and glute.
6. If you feel comfortable and want to deepen the stretch, gently press down on your right knee with your right hand while keeping your chest lifted. If it's comfortable, lean forward slightly to find a deeper stretch.
7. Take slow, deep breaths as you hold the pose, allowing any tension to release.
8. Hold the pose for 30–45 seconds, breathing deeply and consciously.
9. To release, slowly uncross your right leg and place both feet back on the floor.
10. Repeat the pose on the opposite side by crossing your left ankle over your right knee.

Scan the QR code below for the video tutorial

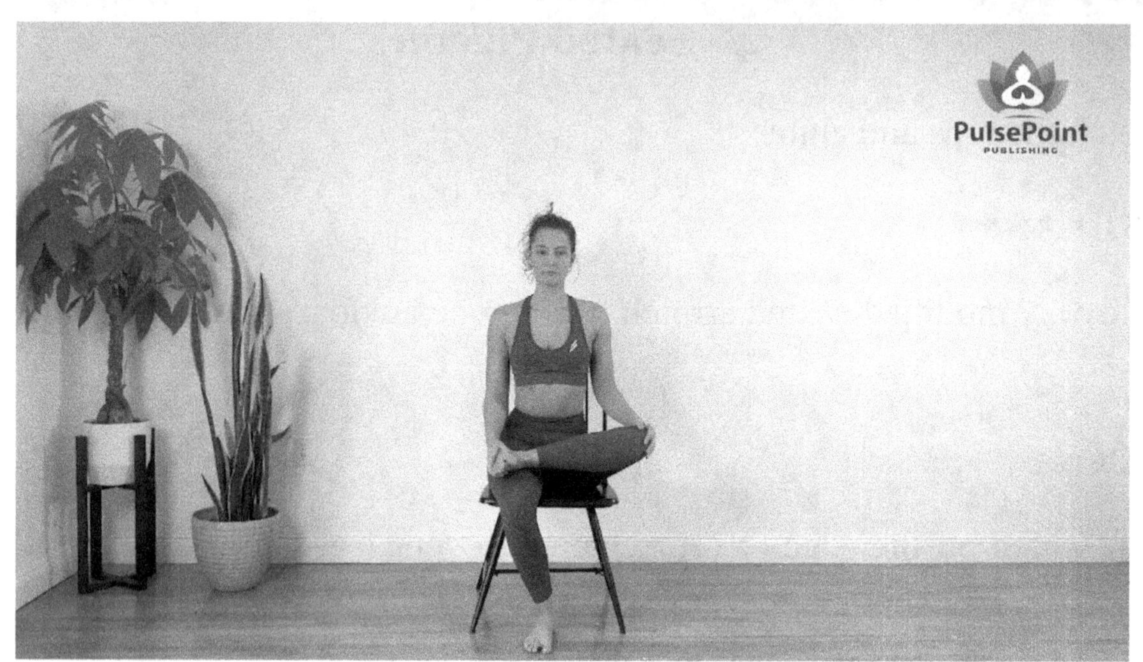

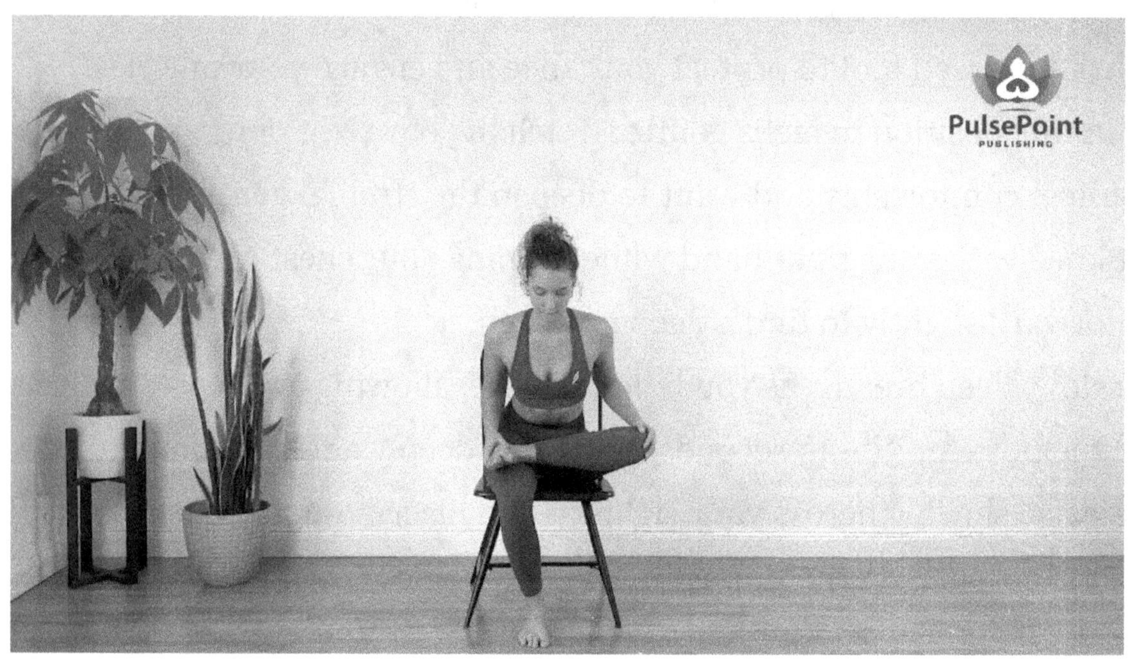

5 - Overhead Shoulder Stretch

Goal: Stretch the shoulders

Difficulty: ★☆☆☆☆

Description: A seated position focusing on extending the arms overhead to stretch and release tension in the shoulders.

Step-by-step:

1. Begin seated comfortably on your chair with your feet flat on the floor, hip-width apart.
2. Sit tall, stretching your spine, and let your shoulders drop away from your ears.
3. Interlace your fingers, pushing your palms out in front of you and then extend them up towards the ceiling.
4. Inhale deeply as you straighten your arms and lift them overhead, extending through your fingertips.
5. Keep your shoulders relaxed and your chest open.
6. If possible, gently tilt your head back slightly to increase the stretch in your shoulders and chest.
7. Hold the pose for 30 seconds, breathing deeply and evenly.
8. Feel the stretch along the sides of your body and through your shoulders.
9. To release, exhale as you lower your arms back down to your sides and release the interlace of your fingers.
10. Repeat 3–5 times.

Scan the QR code below for the video tutorial

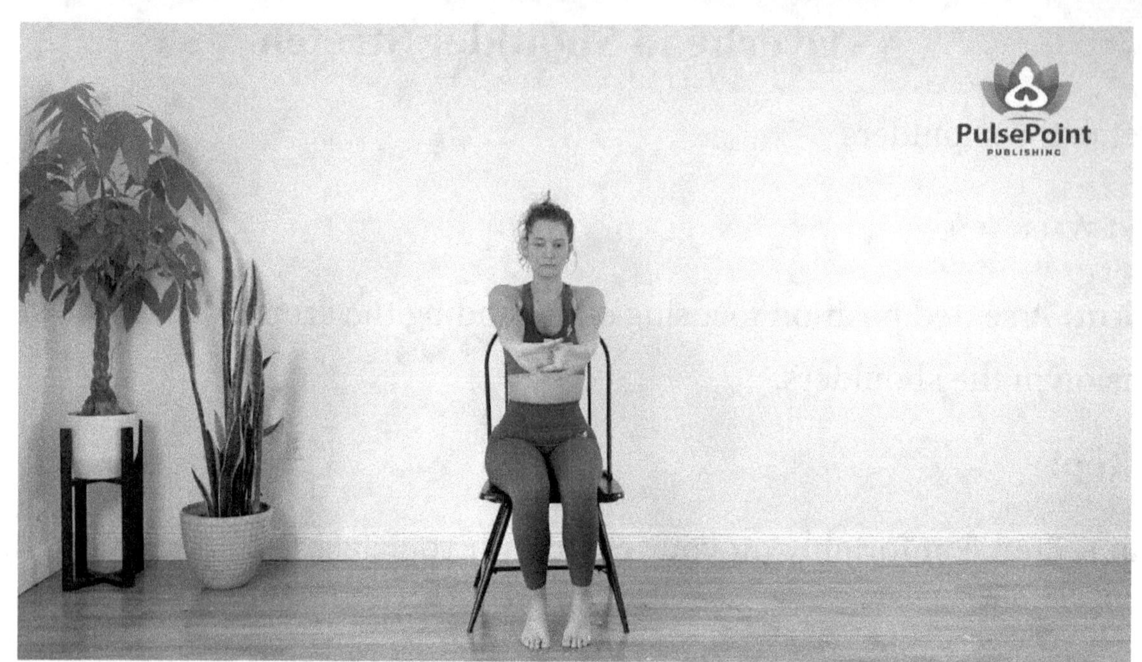

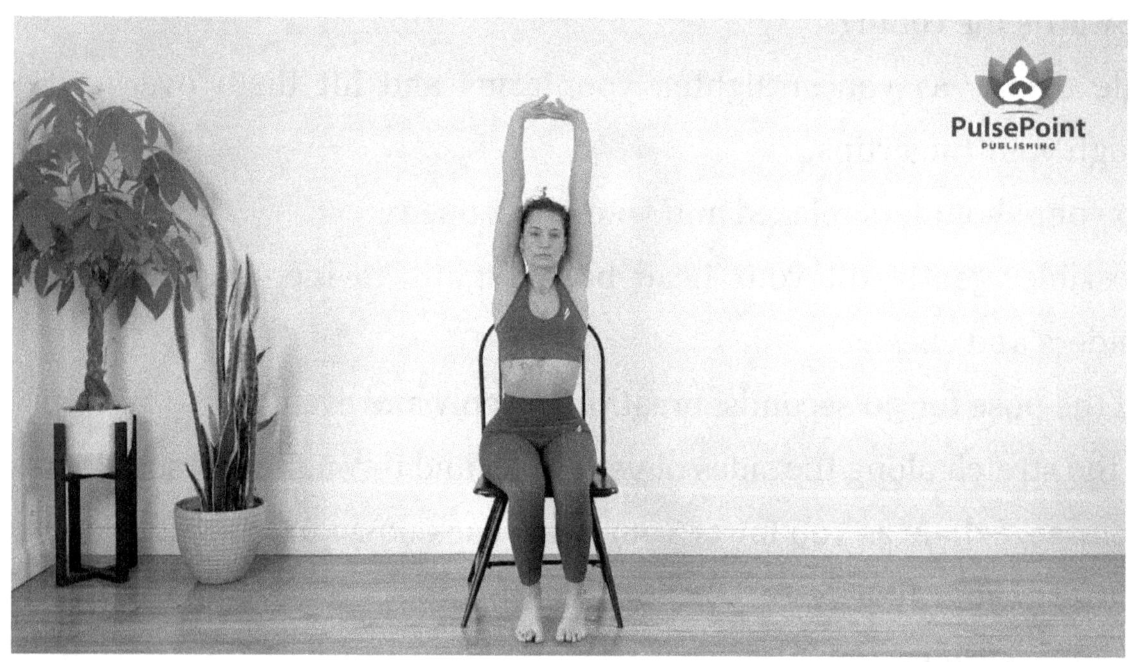

24

6 - Low Lunge - High Lunge

Goal: Strengthen the quads and glutes

Difficulty: ★★★★☆

Description: Transition from a low lunge position, with one foot forward and the other extended back, to a high lunge, creating a seamless flow that enhances strength and stability.

Step-by-step:

1. Begin in a low lunge position.
2. Ensure your front knee is directly above your right ankle and your left leg is at 90 degrees.
3. Keep your hands on your thighs or at the hips for support.
4. Use core muscles to support your body.
5. On an inhale, press firmly into both feet to lift your sit bones off the chair.
6. Exhale, lower the sit bones back down.
7. Keep your gaze forward and lengthen through your spine.
8. Maintain a slight tuck of your tailbone to engage your lower abdominals and protect your lower back.
9. Move through the movement from low lunge to high lunge for 30–60 seconds.
10. Repeat 3–5 times.

Scan the QR code below for the video tutorial

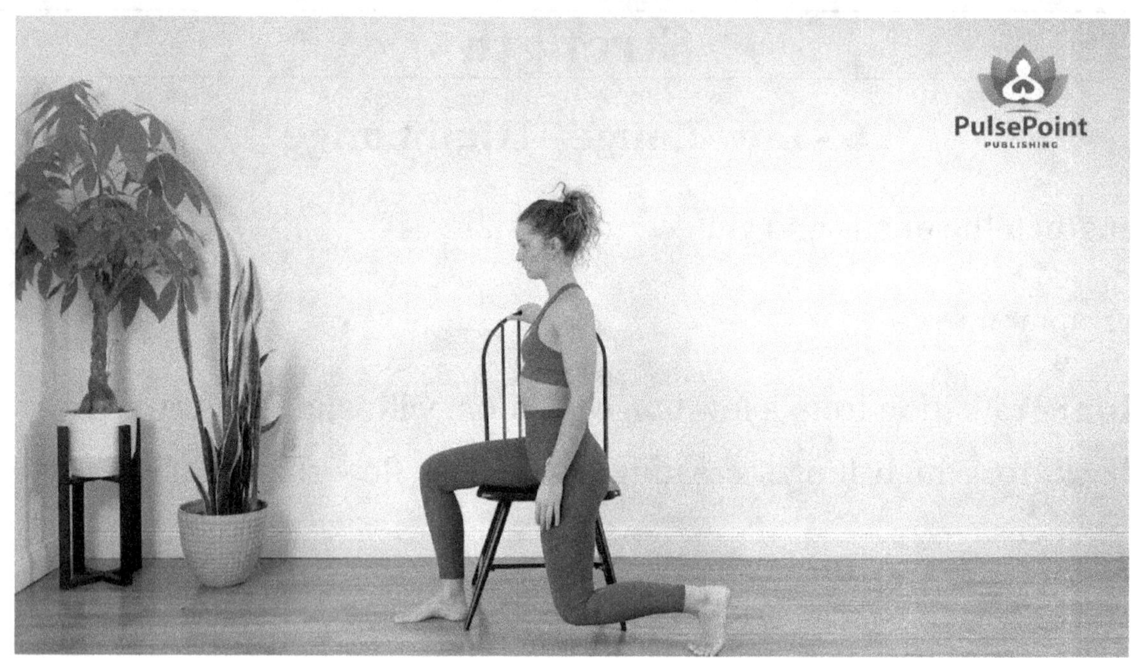

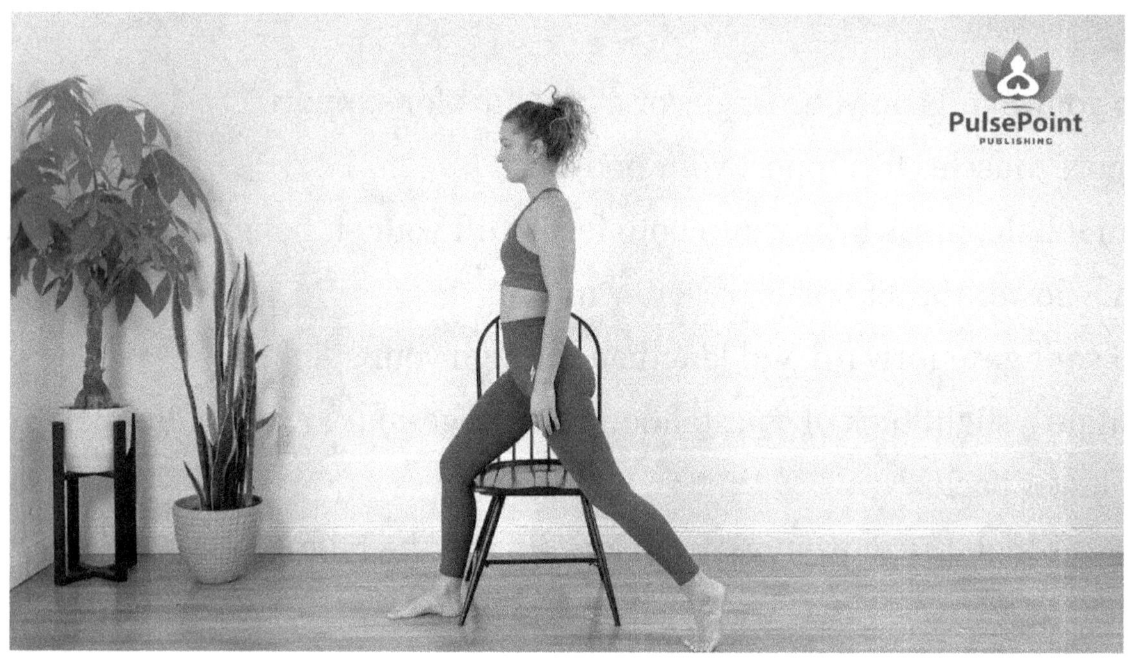

7 - Goddess Lifts

Goal: Strengthen the quads, inners thighs and glutes

Difficulty: ★★★★☆

Description: In a wide-legged squat known as Goddess Pose, push through the feet to lift the sit bones off the chair an inch, engaging the lower body muscles to enhance strength and toning.

Step-by-step:

1. Begin seated comfortably on the edge of your chair with your feet flat on the floor, wider than the hips. Toes pointed outward slightly.
2. Sit up tall, lengthening your spine, and engage your core muscles for stability.
3. Place your hands on your thighs, hold onto the sides of the chair for support, or bring your arms to 90 degrees.
4. Inhale, push through your feet to lift the sit bones off the chair.
5. Exhale, lower back down.
6. Keep your spine long and your chest lifted, maintaining an active and engaged posture.
7. Move through these goddess lifts with your breath for 30–60 seconds.
8. Repeat 3–5 times.

Scan the QR code below for the video tutorial

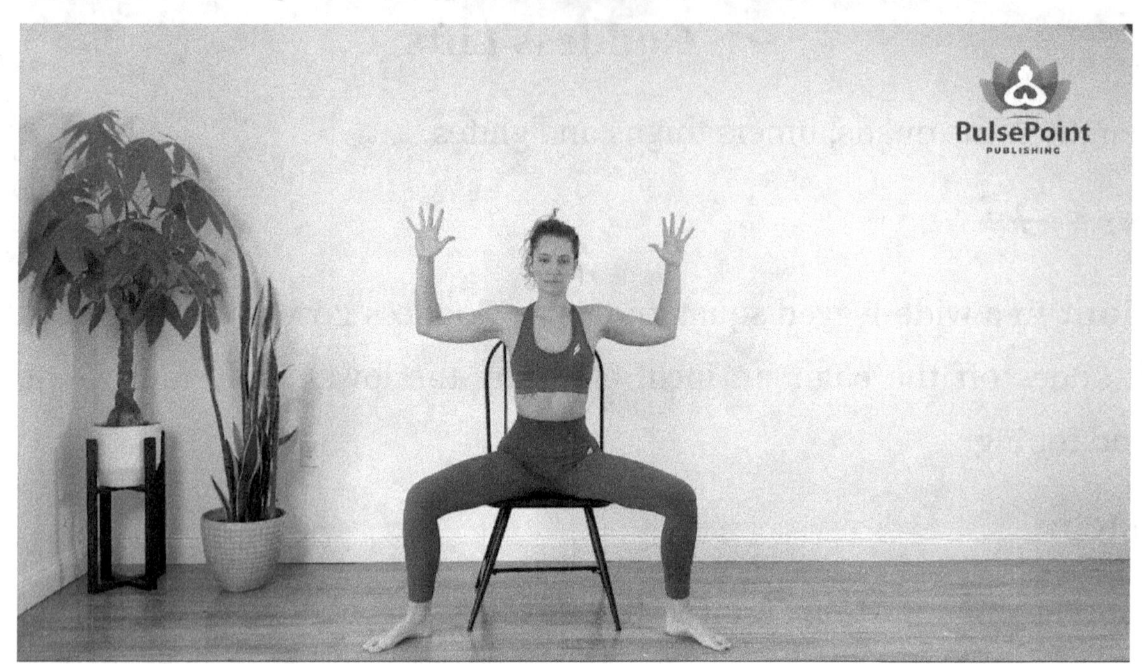

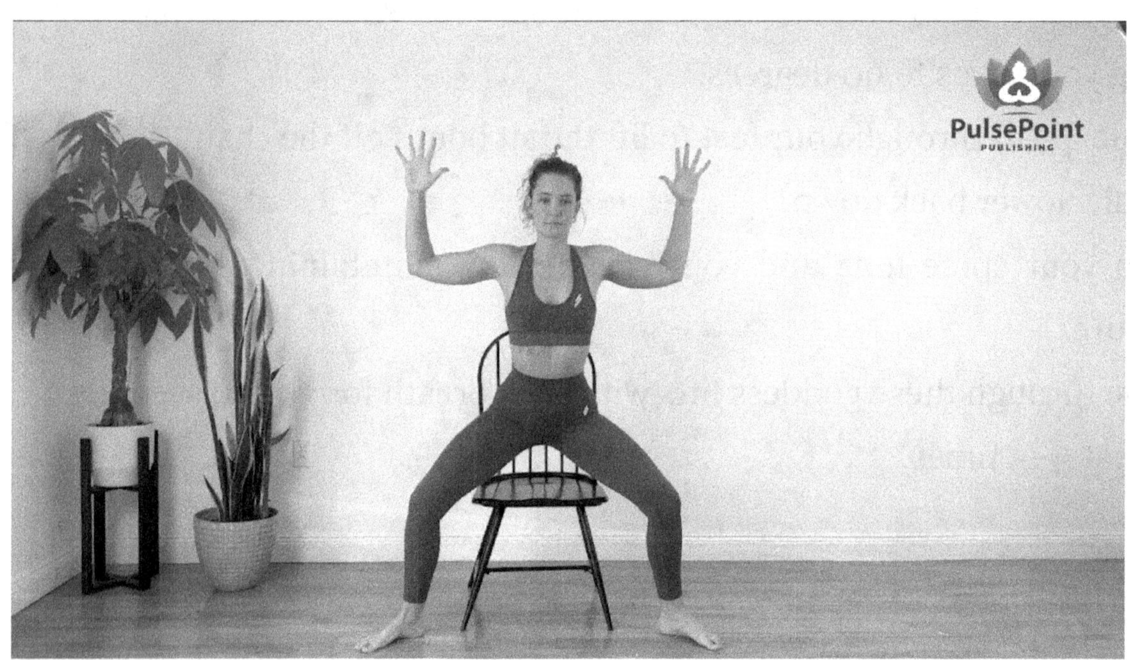

8 - Chair Pose Flow

Goal: Strengthen the quads, glutes, hamstrings, and shoulders

Difficulty: ★★★☆☆

Description: In seated Chair Pose, lean forward and lift the sit bones off the chair an inch, and then sit back down; repeating this process with the breath.

Step-by-step:

1. Begin seated comfortably on the edge of your chair with your feet flat on the floor, hip-width apart.
2. Sit up tall, lengthening your spine, and reach your hands overhead, or on the sides of the chair for support.
3. Take a deep inhale as you engage your core muscles and lift your sit bones slightly off the chair, hovering just above the seat.
4. Keep your knees bent and your feet firmly planted on the floor.
5. On an exhale, slowly lower your sit bones back down onto the chair, maintaining control and stability.
6. Allow your weight to be evenly distributed between your sit bones and feet.
7. Move through this for 30–60 seconds.
8. Repeat 3–5 times.

Scan the QR code below for the video tutorial

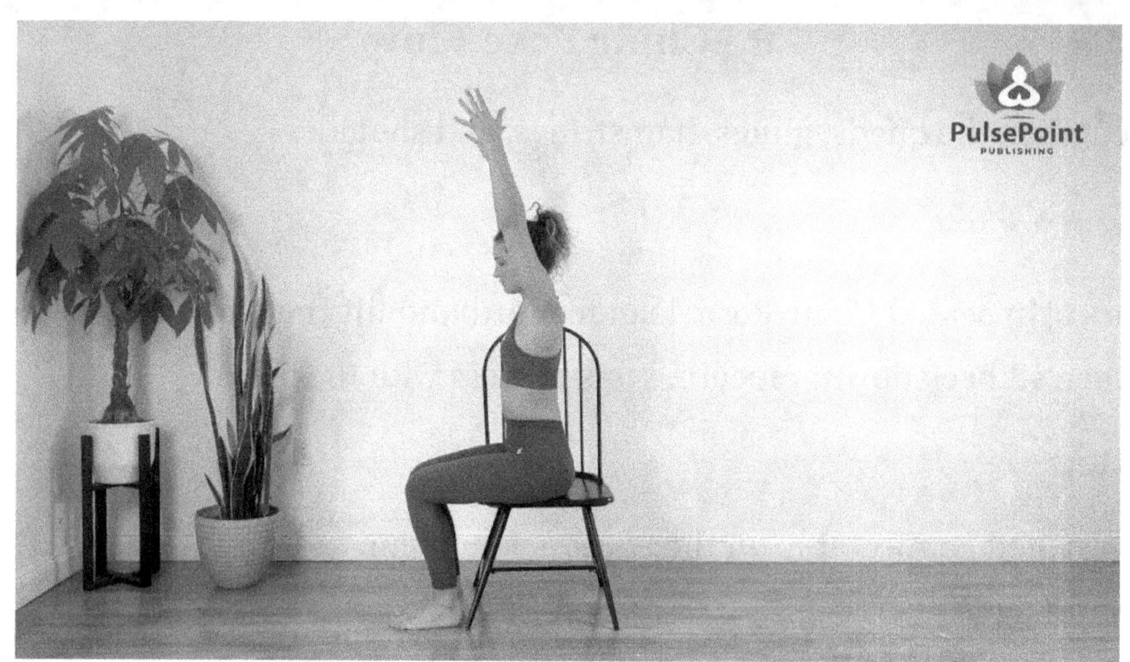

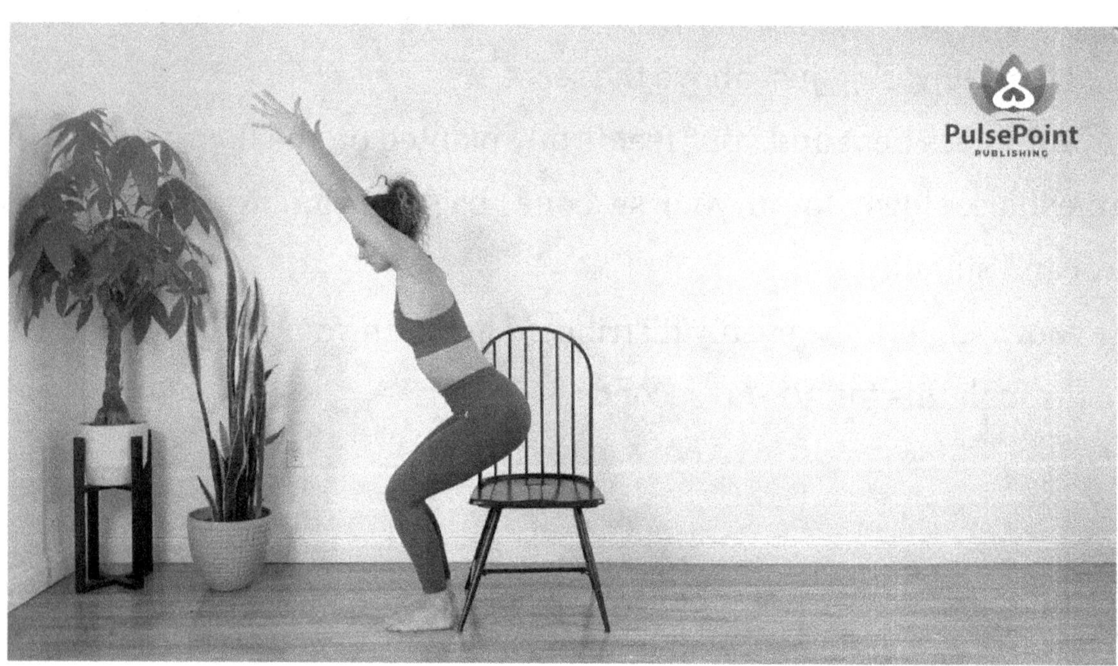

9 - Goddess Side Crunches

Goal: Strengthen the core

Difficulty: ★★☆☆☆

Description: Engage core muscles in a wide-legged seated squat position, incorporating lateral crunches to strengthen and tone the obliques.

Step-by-step:

1. Begin seated comfortably on the edge of your chair with your feet flat on the floor, wider than the hips.
2. Sit up tall, lengthening your spine, and engage your core muscles for stability.
3. Place your hands behind your head, elbows extended out to the sides.
4. Inhale to prepare.
5. Exhale and tilt your torso to the right, bringing your right elbow to your right thigh.
6. Simultaneously, engage your obliques to crunch your right ribcage towards your right hip.
7. Inhale to return to the center, lengthening your spine.
8. Exhale as you tilt your torso to the left, bringing your left elbow towards your left thigh while crunching your left ribcage towards your left hip.
9. Flow between the two sides while harmonizing your breath with the action.
10. Move through this for 30–60 seconds.
11. Repeated 3–5 times.

Scan the QR code below for the video tutorial

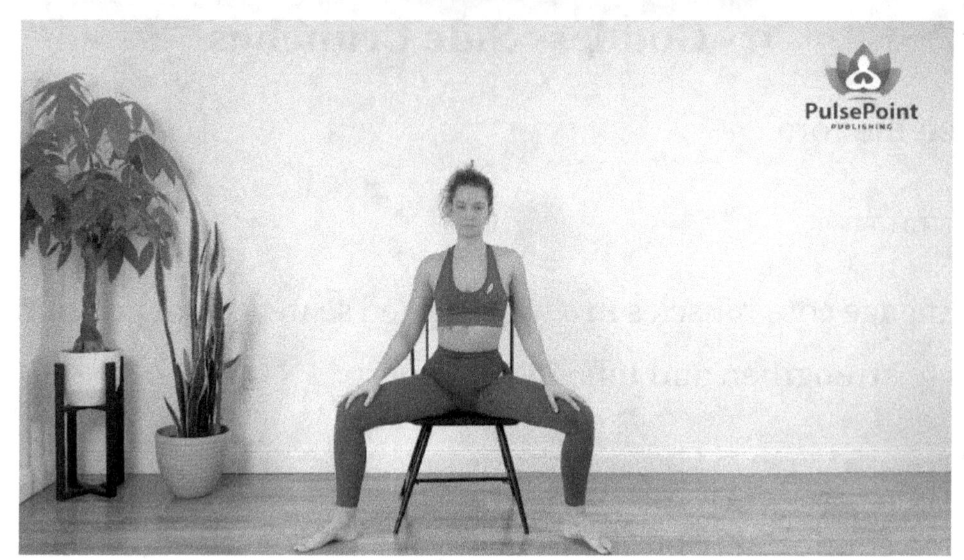

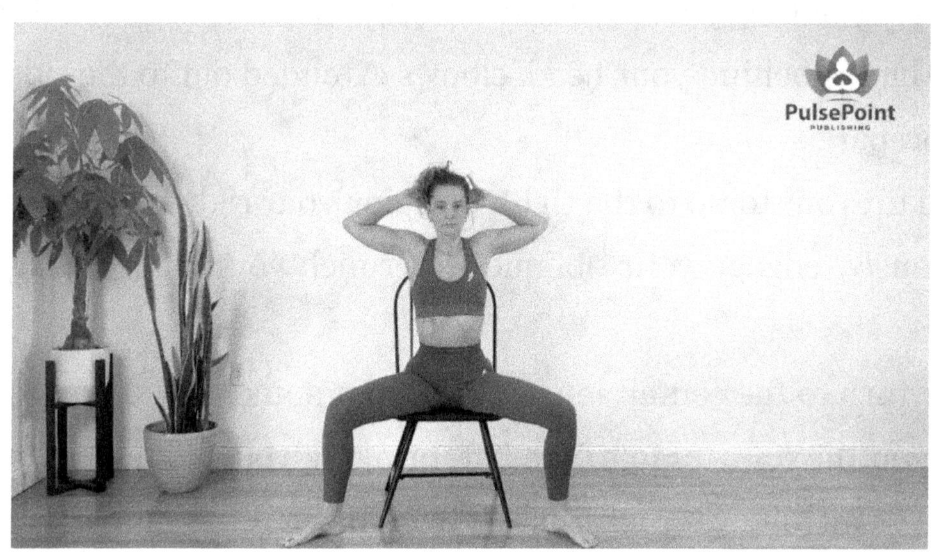

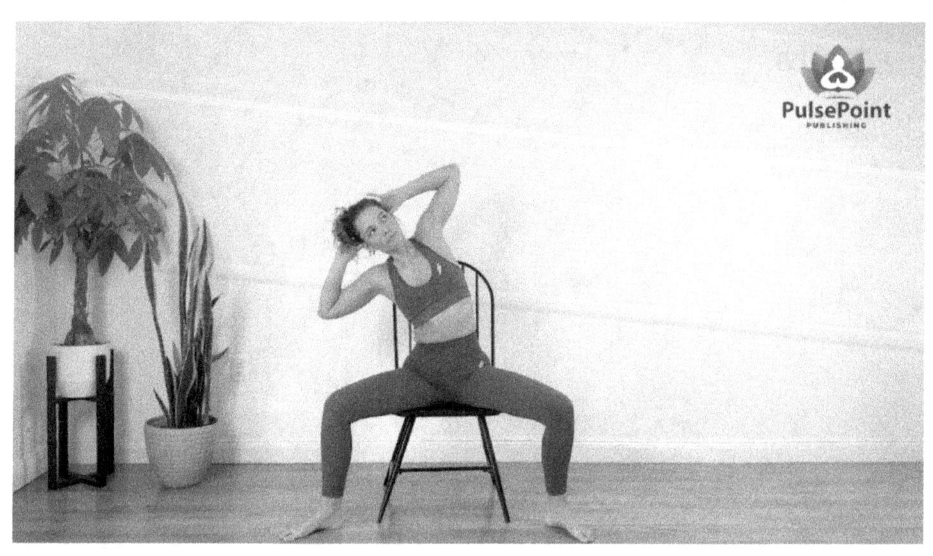

10 - Warrior III Crunches

Goal: Strengthen the quads, glutes, and core

Difficulty: ★★★★☆

Description: Balancing on one leg in a Warrior III position, integrate core crunches to enhance abdominal strength and stability.

Step-by-step:

1. Begin standing facing the chair, place one hand on the back of the chair for support.
2. Stand up tall, lengthening your spine, begin to lean forward as you keep one foot grounded, and the other foot floats up behind you.
3. Move your hands to the seat of your chair.
4. Attempting to create a 'T' shape with your body, lengthening from your lifted heel, all the way up your spine.
5. Use core muscles to support your body.
6. Inhale, draw your lifted knee towards your heart as you round the spine.
7. Exhale, extend your leg back out behind you.
8. As you move, keep your right hip level with your left hip and your hips squared towards the front of the chair.
9. Move through this movement for 30–60 seconds.
10. Repeat 3–5 times.
11. After completing the desired number of repetitions, switch sides.

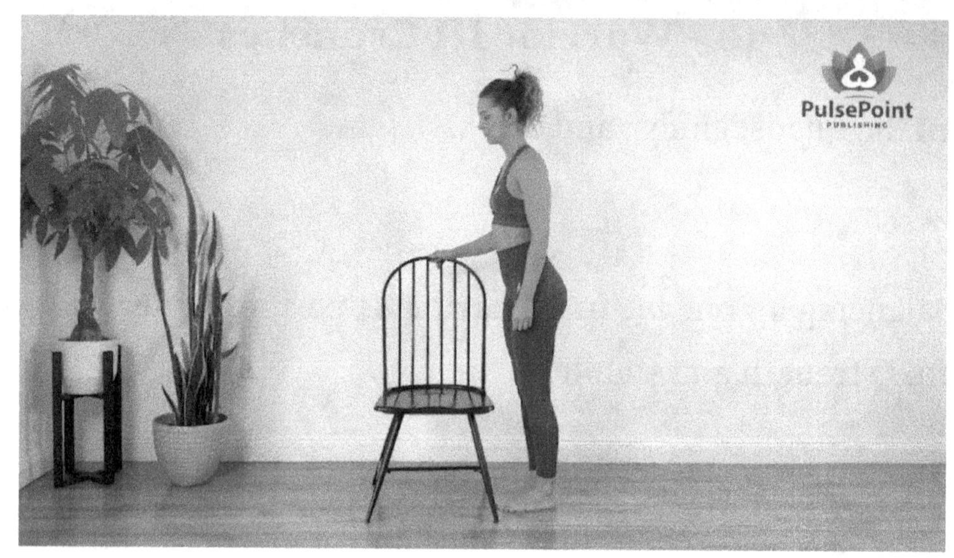

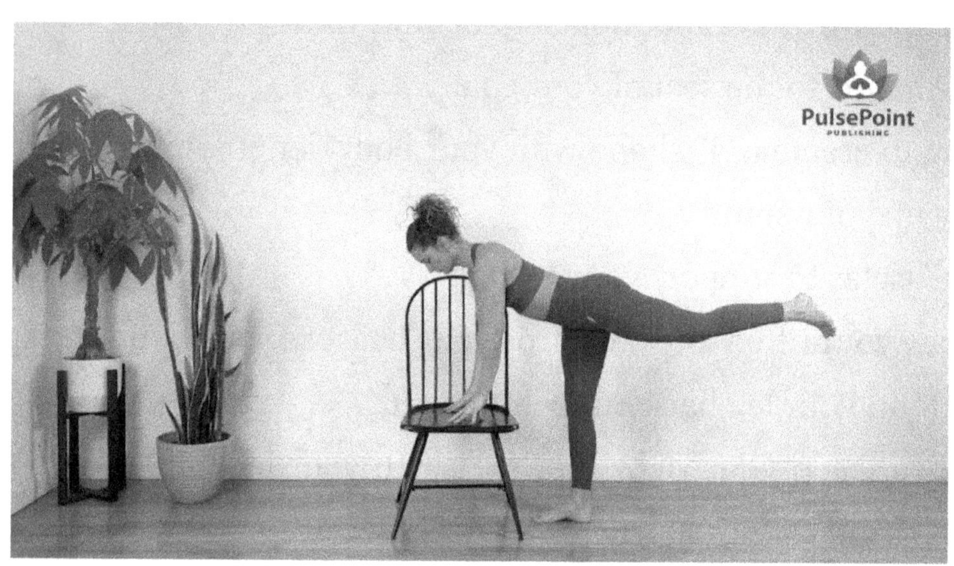

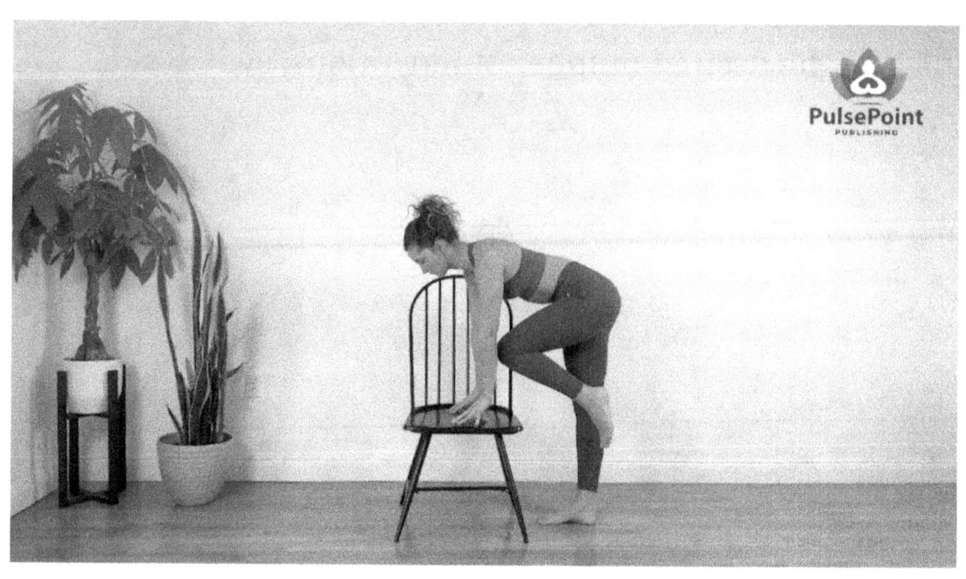

11 - Palm Tree

Goal: Balance on standing leg, lengthen the spine, strengthen stabilizer muscles

Difficulty: ★☆☆☆☆

Description: A standing yoga pose where one arm is extended overhead while standing on the balls of the feet, promoting lengthening, and stretching through the entire body.

Step-by-step:

1. Stand facing the chair with feet hips width apart.
2. Stand tall, stretching your spine, and lowering your shoulders away from your ears.
3. Use one hand to hold the back of the chair and extend the other arm up to the ceiling.
4. Inhale deeply to lengthen through your spine and lift onto the balls of both feet.
5. Hold the stretch for 30–60 seconds, breathing deeply and evenly.
6. Bring the heels back to the floor, and switch arms.
7. Repeat 3–5 times on each side.

Scan the QR code below for the video tutorial

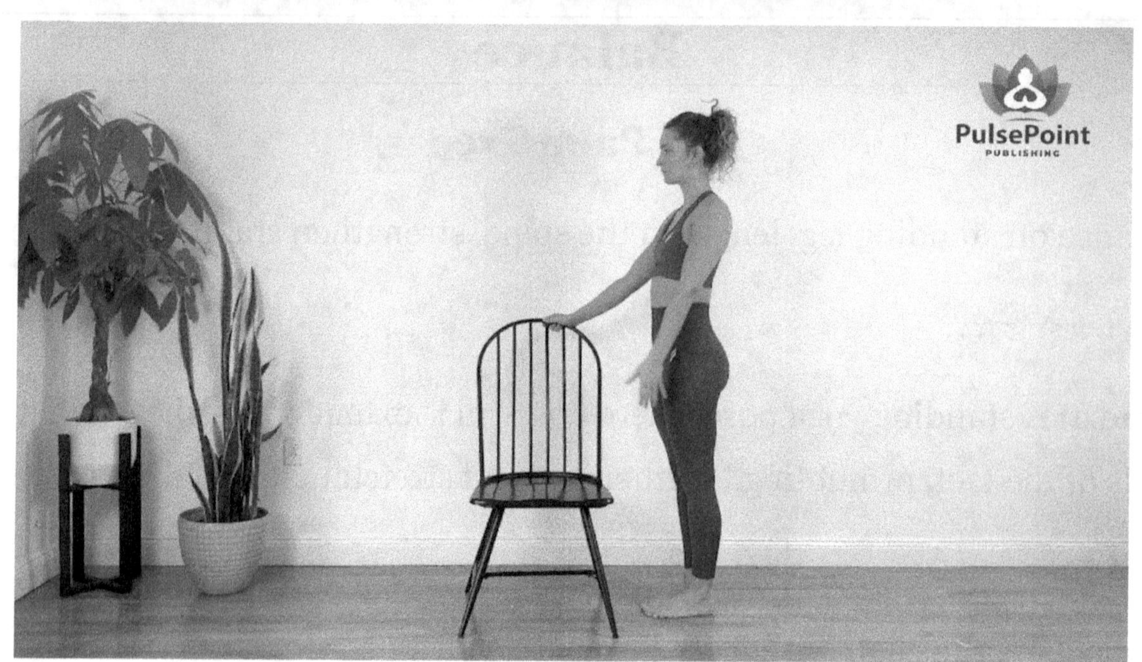

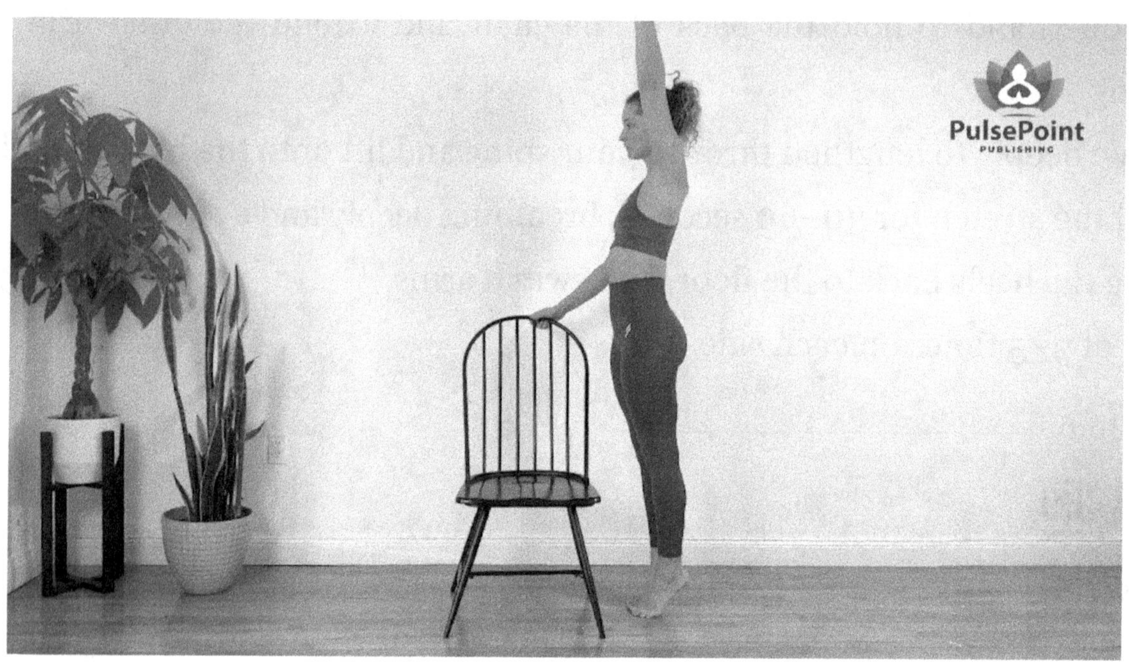

12 - Standing Low Lunge Half Split

Goal: Balance on standing leg, strengthen the quads and hamstrings

Difficulty: ★★★★☆

Description: Transition from a standing lunge position into a half split, moving back and forth with the breath.

Step-by-step:

1. Begin standing beside your chair with your feet hip-width apart, facing the chair for support.
2. Hold onto the back of the chair with one hand for stability.
3. Step one foot back on the seat of the chair, allowing the knee to bend, creating a 90-degree angle.
4. Keep your hips squared towards the chair to maintain proper alignment.
5. With an inhale, straighten the lifted leg into half split. Place the heel on the seat of the chair and keep the foot flexed.
6. Exhale, move the leg back to 90 degrees in the standing low lunge position.
7. Continue moving back and forth following your breath.
8. Find movement for 30–60 seconds, and then switch sides.
9. Repeat 3–5 times.

Scan the QR code below for the video tutorial

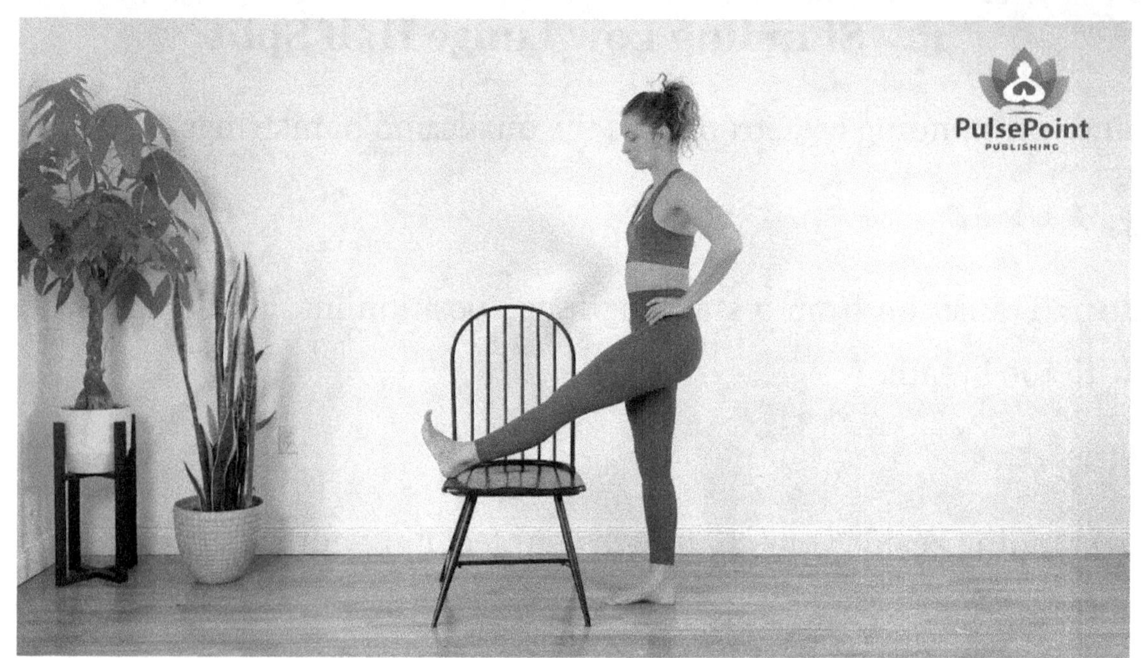

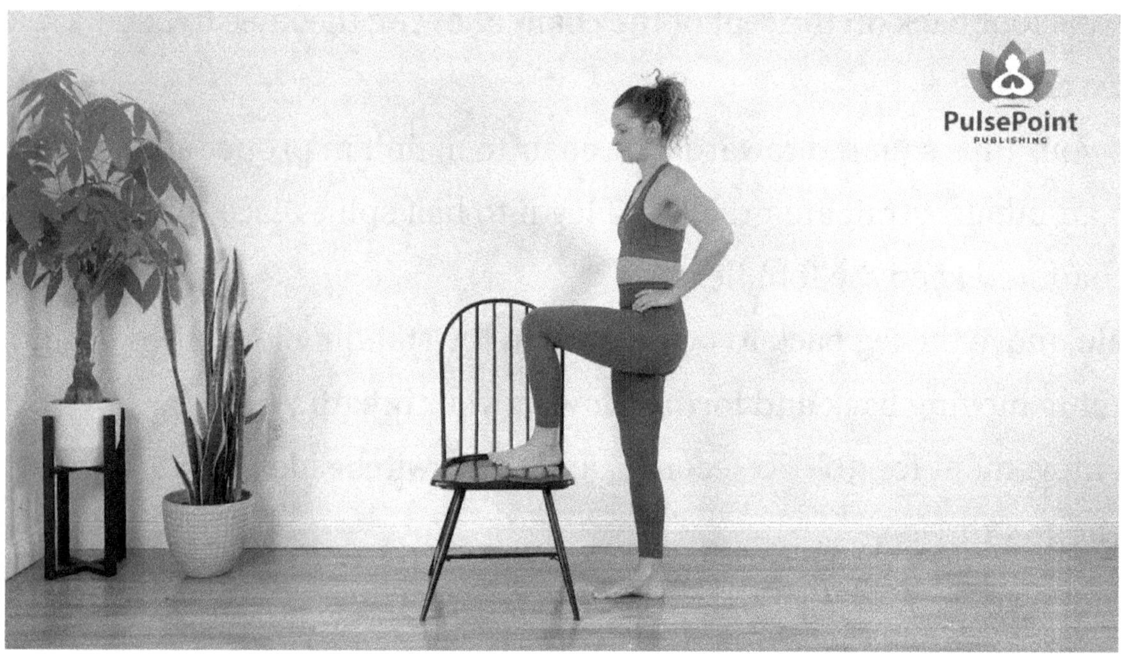

13 - Tree Pose

Goal: Balance on standing leg, strengthen the core, and open the hips

Difficulty: ★★☆☆☆

Description: A standing yoga pose involving balancing on one leg with the other foot placed on the inner thigh, calf, or ankle, promoting stability and concentration.

Step-by-step:

1. Stand next to your chair, feet, hip-width apart.
2. Sit up straight, extending your spine and using your core muscles for stability.
3. Shift your weight onto your inside foot and firmly press it into the floor.
4. Bend the opposite leg slightly, externally rotate your knee.
5. Bring your foot to the inside of your ankle to a kickstand position with the heel resting gently on your leg as the ball of the foot is rested on the ground.
6. One step further, bring your foot to the inside of your shin.
7. If you wish to take it further, bring your foot to the inside of your thigh.
8. Keep one hand on the chair for support.
9. Find a focal point in front of you to help maintain balance and concentration.
10. Hold the pose for 30–60 seconds, breathing deeply and evenly.
11. Repeat on the other side.
12. Repeat 3–5 times.

Scan the QR code below for the video tutorial

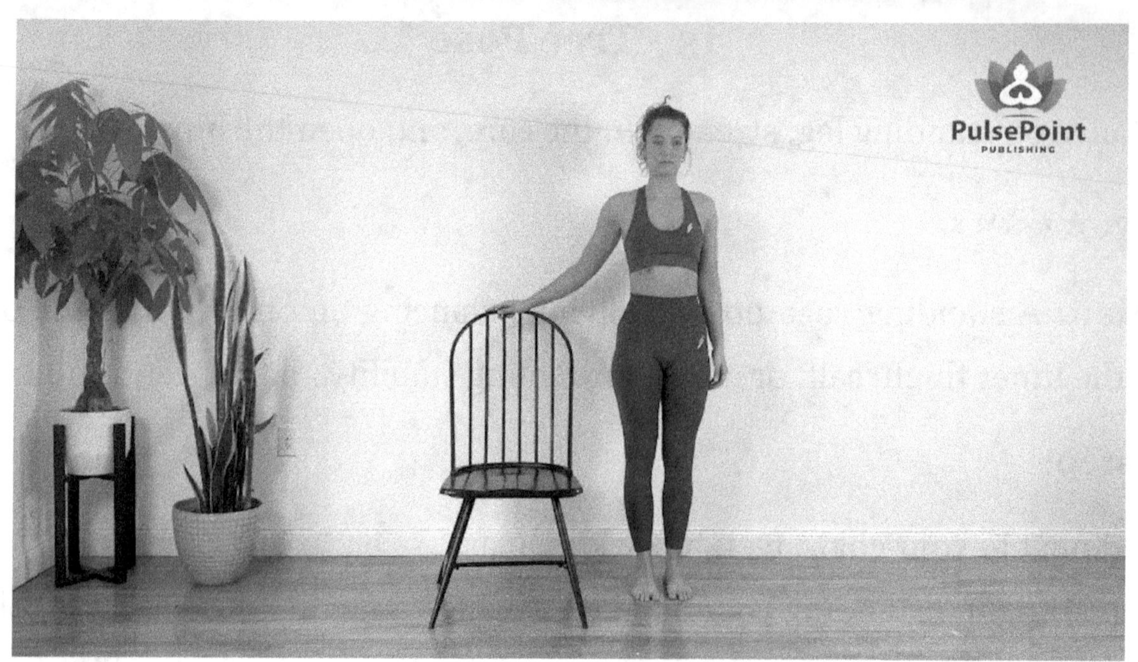

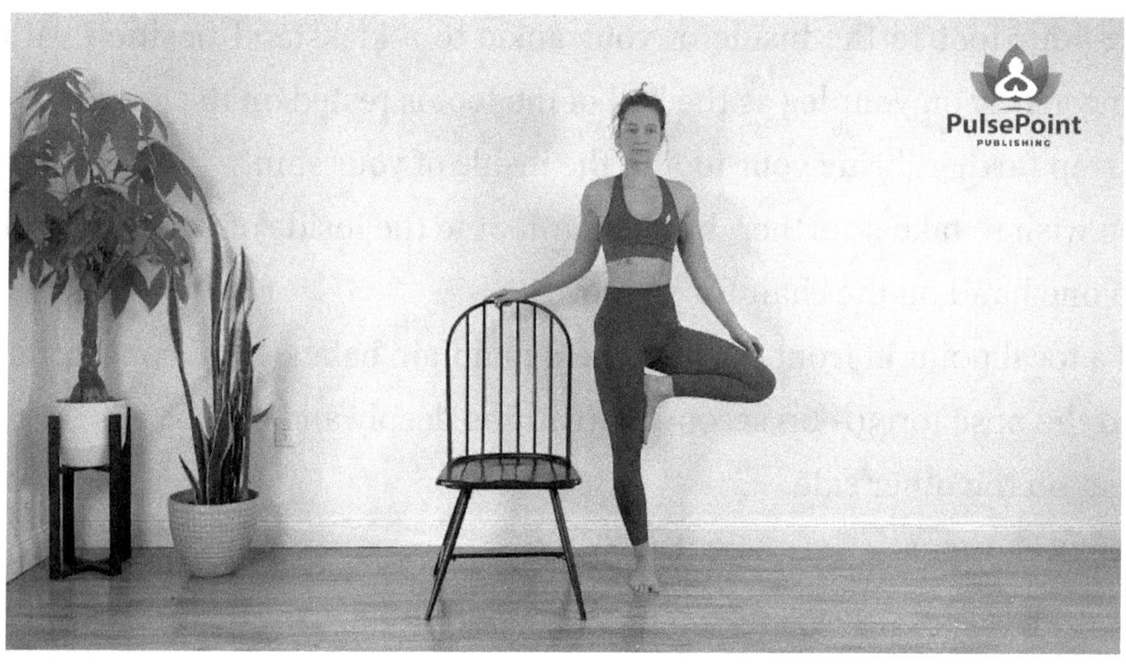

14 - Stork Bird

Goal: Balance on standing leg, strengthen the core, and strengthen stabilizer muscles

Difficulty: ★★☆☆☆

Description: A standing yoga pose where one knee is lifted, while extending the foot, enhancing balance and focus.

Step-by-step:

1. Stand next to your chair, feet, hip-width apart.
2. Sit up tall, lengthening your spine, and engage your core muscles for stability.
3. Shift your weight onto one foot and firmly press it into the floor.
4. Lift the opposite knee up towards the ceiling.
5. Extended your foot, pointing the toes towards the ground.
6. Keep one hand on the chair for support.
7. Find a focal point in front of you to help maintain balance and concentration.
8. Hold for 30–60 seconds and repeat on the other side.
9. Repeat 3–5 times.

Scan the QR code below for the video tutorial

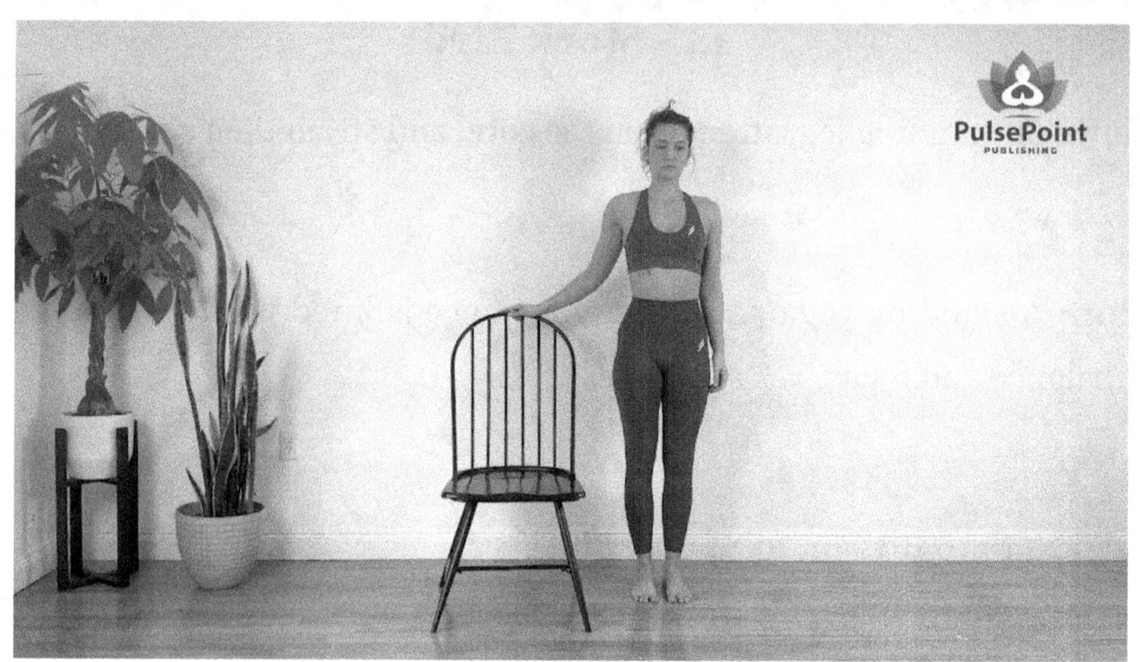

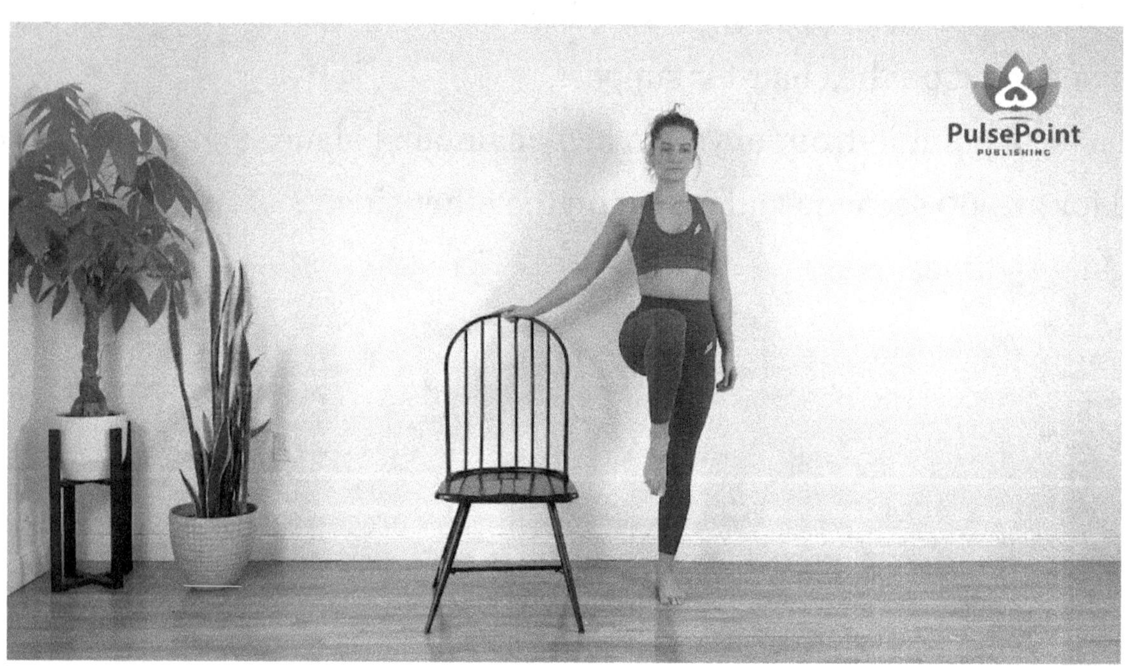

15 - Warrior III

Goal: Balance on standing leg, strengthen quads and glutes, and strengthen stabilizer muscles

Difficulty: ★★★★☆

Description: A standing pose that involves balancing on one leg while extending the other leg backward and parallel to the ground, focusing on strength and stability.

Step-by-step:

1. Stand facing the chair with your feet hip-width apart, toes pointing forward.
2. Place one hand lightly on the back of the chair for support, ensuring a firm grip.
3. Engage your core muscles to keep your body stable and balanced.
4. Shift your weight onto your left foot and firmly press it into the floor.
5. Slowly lift one foot off the ground, bringing it straight back behind you.
6. Keep your right leg parallel to the floor, toes pointing down towards the ground.
7. Ensure your hips are squared towards the chair to maintain proper alignment.
8. Lengthen through your spine, keeping your torso parallel to the floor.
9. Place your hands on the seat of the chair for support. Maintain a comfortable shoulder position away from your ears, with your chest wide.
10. Hold the pose for 30–60 seconds, breathing deeply and evenly.
11. Repeat on the other side.
12. Repeat 3–5 times.

Scan the QR code below for the video tutorial

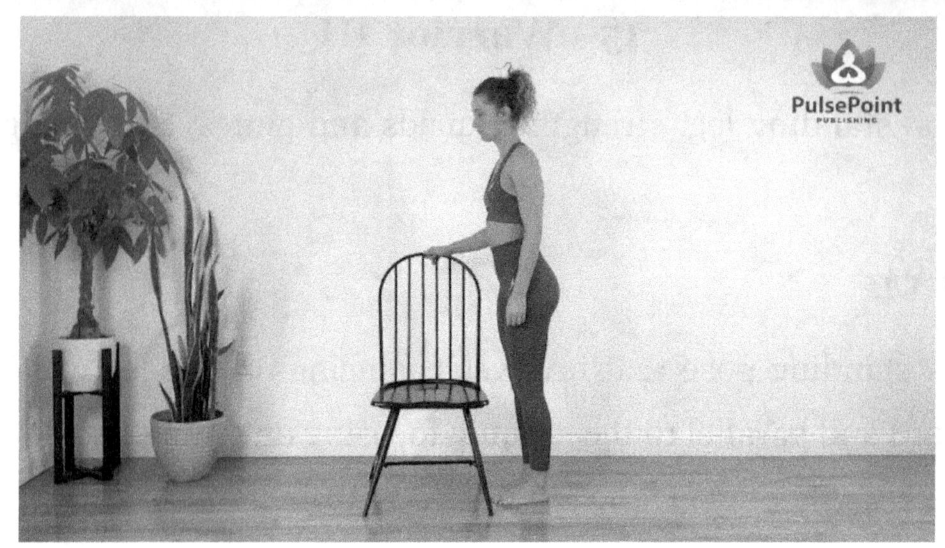

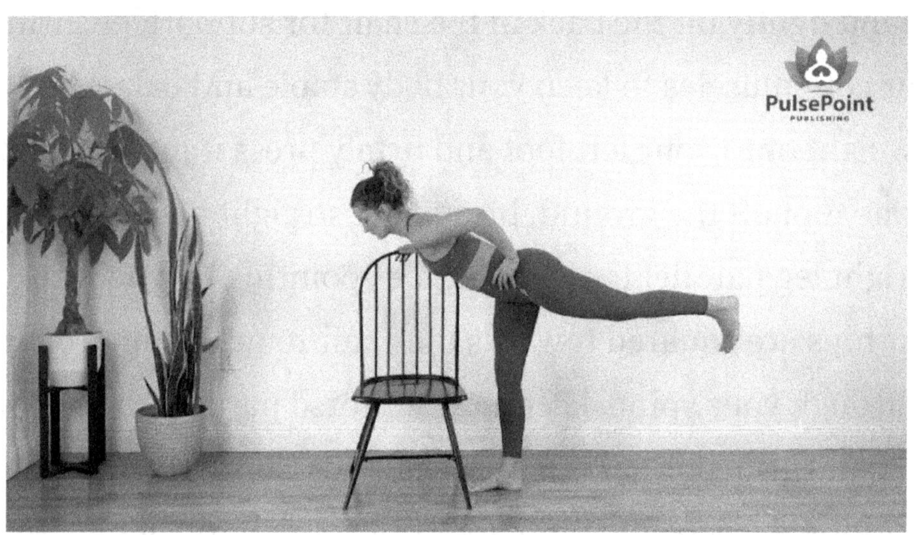

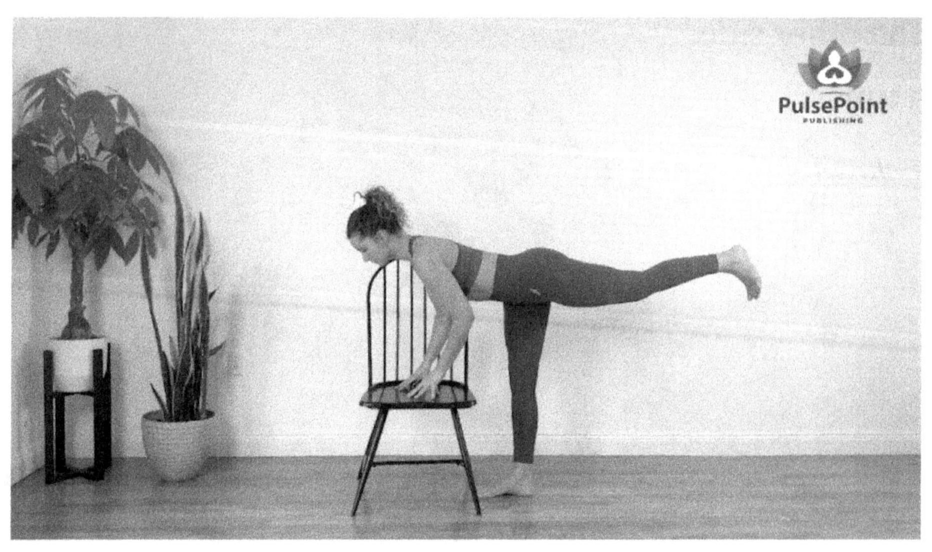

16 - Triangle Arm Rotations

Goal: Develop mobility through the shoulders

Difficulty: ★★★★☆

Description: While in a Triangle pose, incorporate rotating arm movements to enhance shoulder flexibility and promote a dynamic stretch through the torso and arms.

Step-by-step:

1. Stand beside the chair with your feet wide apart, wider than hip-width distance. Place with front foot facing forward, the back foot at 90 degrees with hips externally rotated.
2. Place one hand on the seat of the chair in front of you; the same side arm as the front foot.
3. Extend your second arm towards the ceiling while maintaining it in line with your shoulder.
4. Inhale deeply to lengthen through your spine and engage your core muscles.
5. Exhale as you sweep your lifted arm towards the chair.
6. Inhale, rotate your arm back towards the ceiling.
7. Exhale, unwind.
8. Through this movement maintain the length in your spine, avoiding rounding or collapsing.
9. Continue the arm rotations for several breaths, feeling a gentle opening and release in your shoulder and upper back.
10. Move through this for 30–60 seconds.
11. Repeat the pose on the opposite side.
12. Repeat each side 3–5 times.

Scan the QR code for the video tutorial

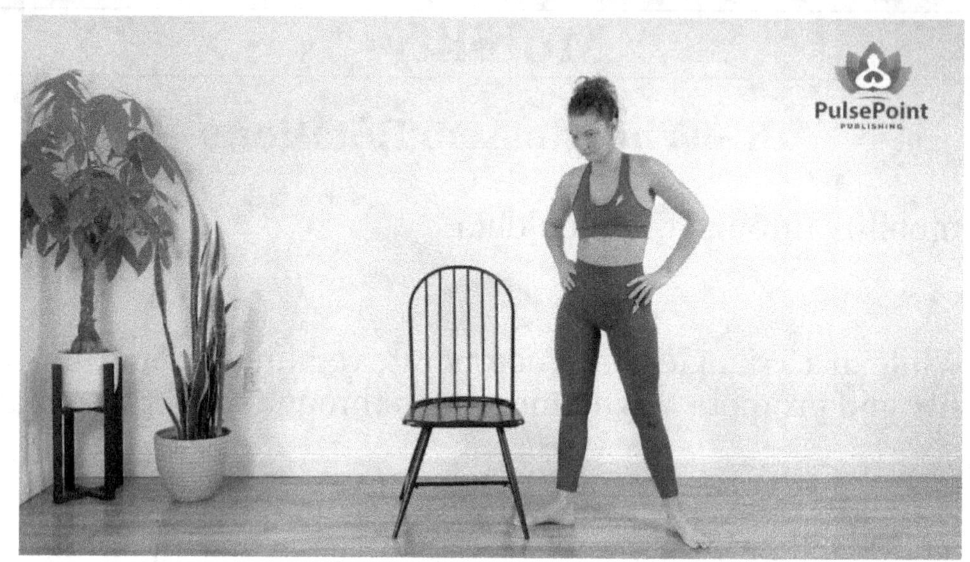

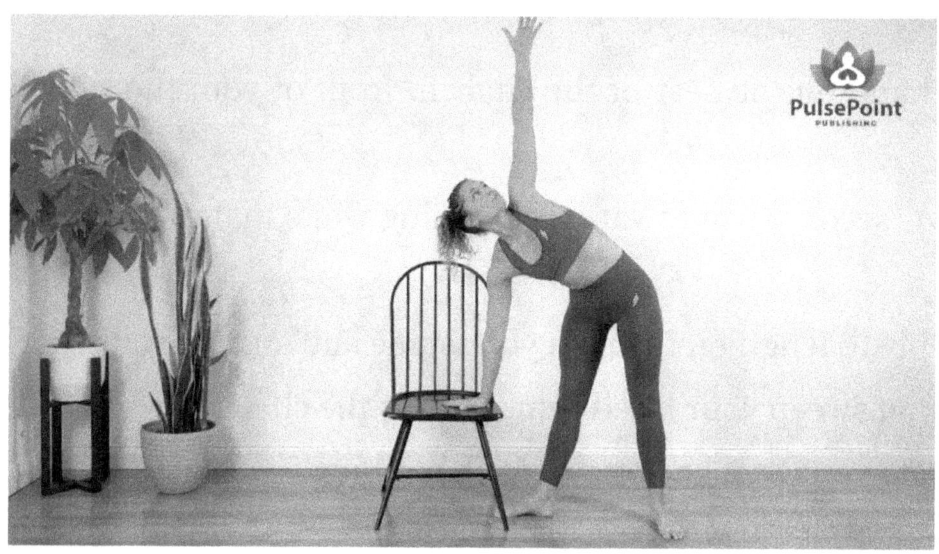

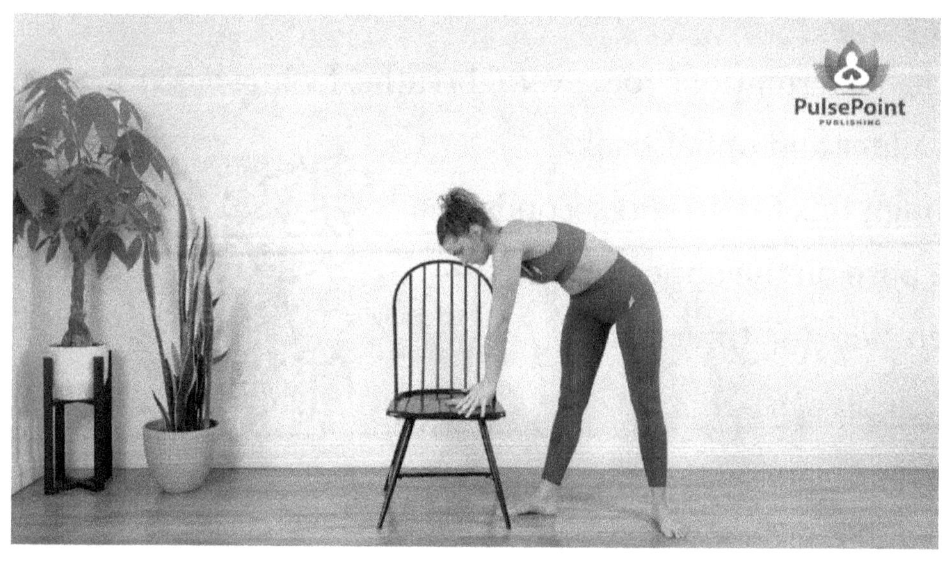

17 - Seated Cat/Cow

Goal: Develop mobility through the spine

Difficulty: ★☆☆☆☆

Description: A seated variation of the traditional Cat/Cow Pose, involving spinal flexion and extension while seated to enhance flexibility and release tension.

Step-by-step:

1. Begin seated comfortably on the edge of your chair with your feet flat on the floor, hip-width apart.
2. Sit up tall, lengthening your spine, and place your hands on your thighs or knees for support.
3. Inhale deeply and arch your back, lifting your chest and tilting your pelvis forward, coming into Cow Pose.
4. Allow your belly to gently drop towards the floor, creating a slight backbend.
5. Lift your gaze towards the ceiling, opening through your chest and shoulders.
6. Hold the Cow Pose for a moment, feeling a stretch through your abdomen and front body.
7. Exhale slowly as you round your spine, tucking your chin towards your chest and drawing your belly button towards your spine, coming into Cat Pose.
8. Press your hands into your thighs or knees as you round your back, creating space between your shoulder blades.
9. Drop your head and let it hang heavy, releasing any tension in your neck.
10. Hold the Cat Pose for a moment, feeling a stretch through your upper back and shoulders.
11. Continue to flow between Seated Cow (inhale) and Seated Cat (exhale), synchronizing your breath with the movement.
12. Repeat the sequence for 30–60 seconds.
13. Repeat 3–5 times.

Scan the QR code for the video tutorial

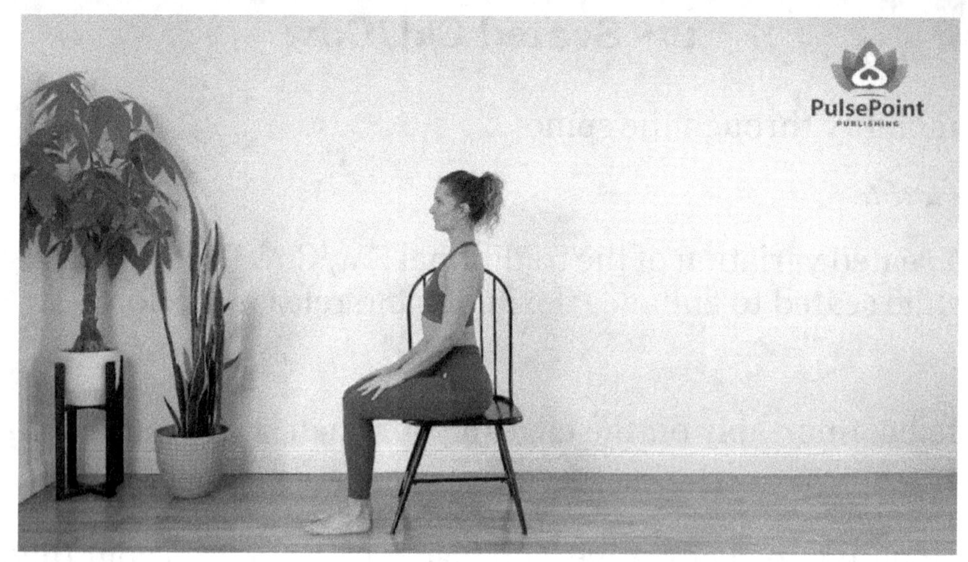

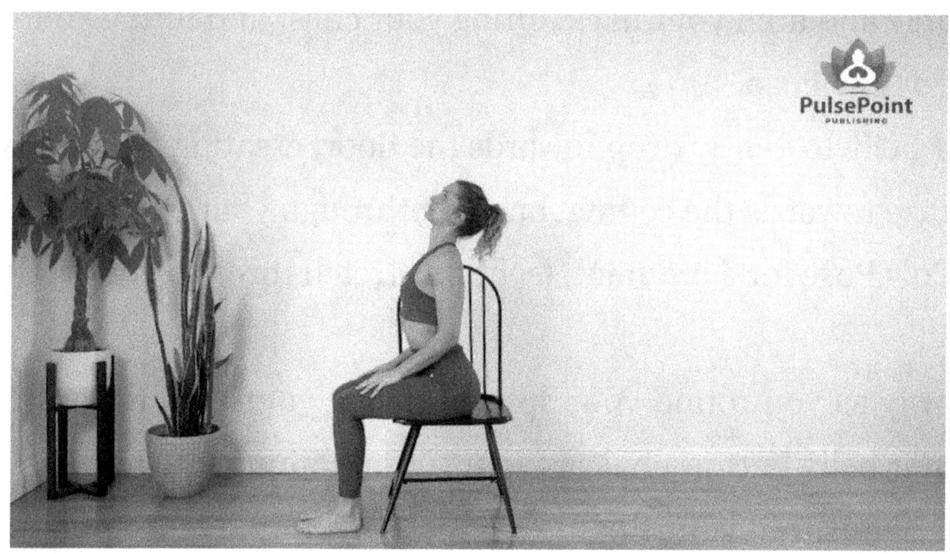

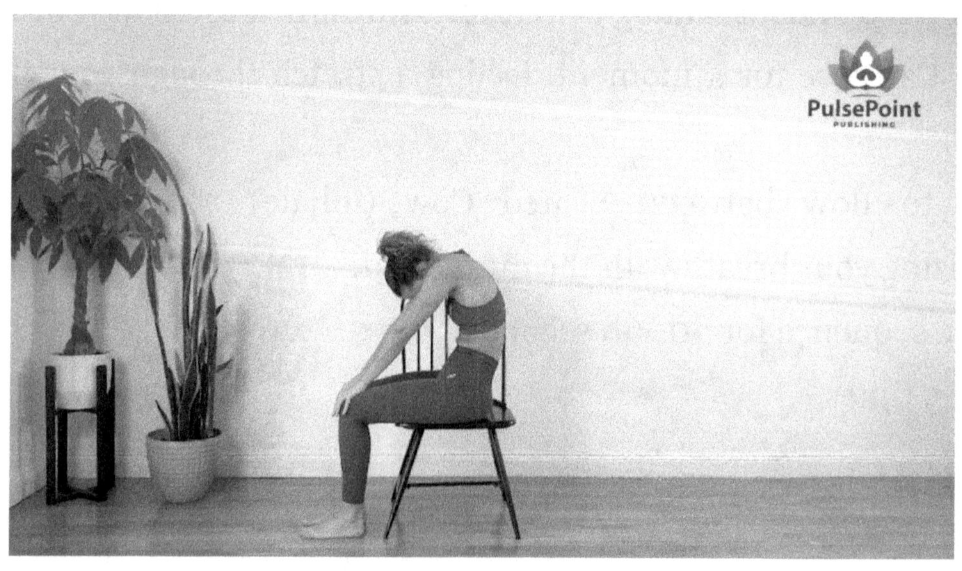

18 - Seated Twist

Goal: Develop mobility through the shoulders and the spine

Difficulty: ★★☆☆☆

Description: A seated position incorporating a twist of the torso to stretch and strengthen the spine, promoting flexibility and improved range of motion.

Step-by-step:

1. Begin seated comfortably on the edge of your chair with your feet flat on the floor, hip-width apart.
2. Sit up tall, lengthening your spine, and place your hands on your thighs or the sides of the chair for support.
3. Inhale deeply to lengthen through your spine, reach your hands overhead.
4. Exhale to gently twist your torso to one side.
5. Place one hand on the back of the chair or the side of the chair seat for support.
6. Bring your other hand to the outside of your right thigh or knee.
7. Use your left hand to gently guide your torso deeper into the twist, without forcing or straining.
8. Keep your chest up and your shoulders loose, away from your ears.
9. Lengthen through the crown of your head as you twist, maintaining a tall spine.
10. Gaze over your shoulder if comfortable or keep your gaze forward for a gentler variation.
11. Hold the twist for 30–60 seconds, breathing deeply and evenly.
12. Repeat the twist on the opposite side by twisting your torso to the left.
13. Repeat 3–5 times on each side.

Scan the QR code below for the video tutorial

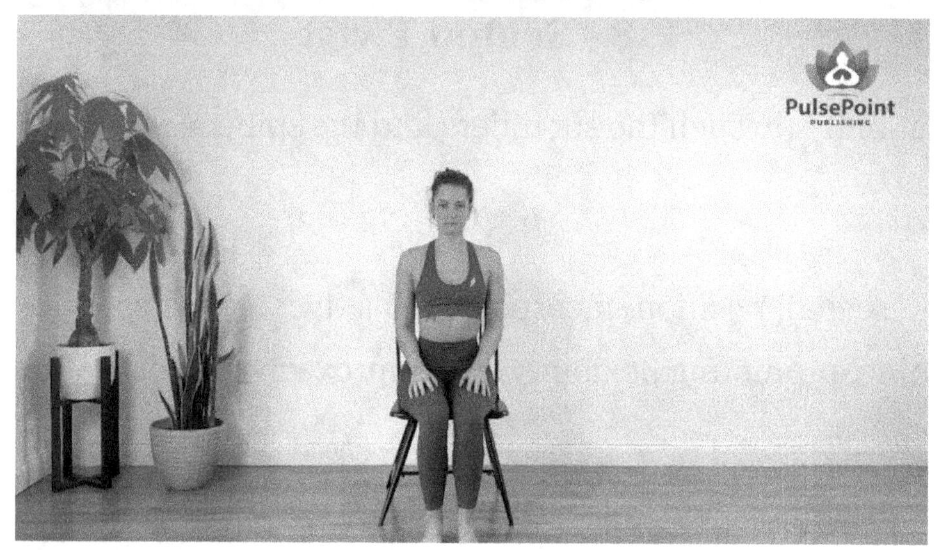

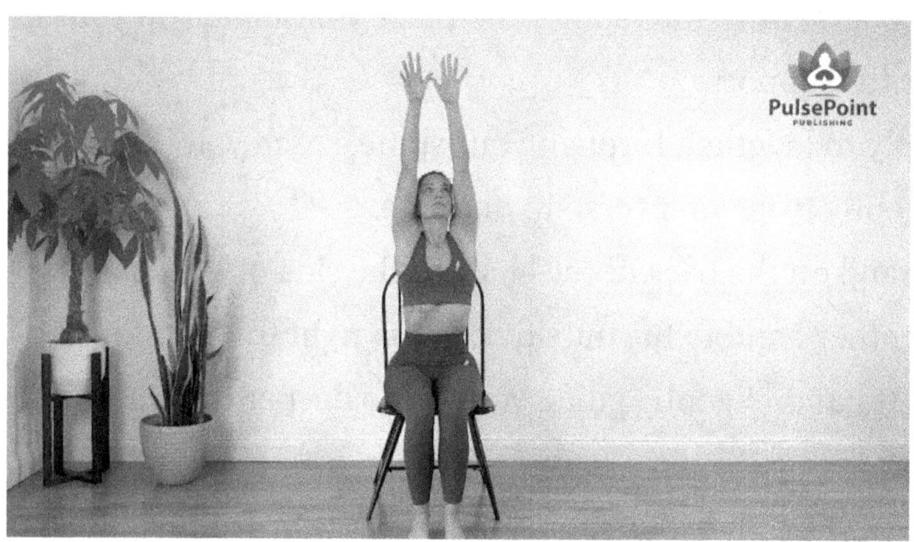

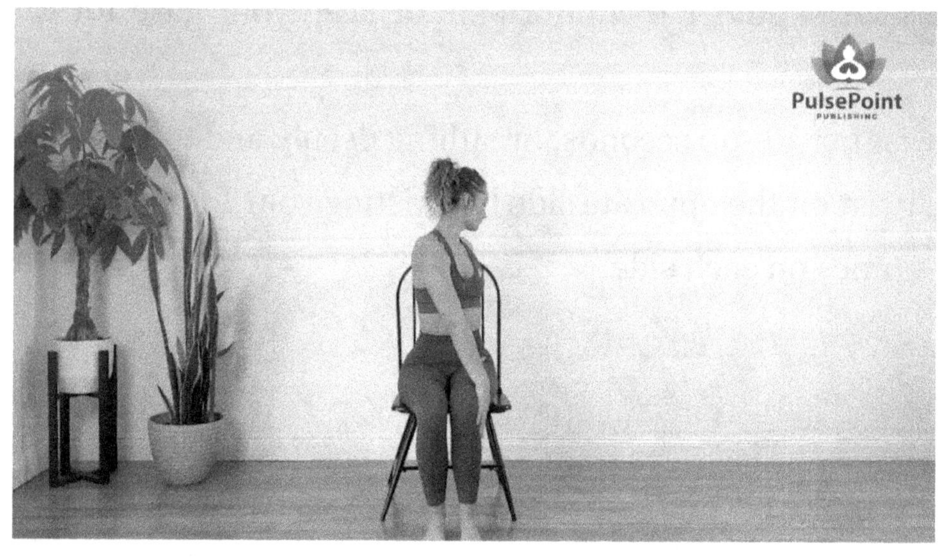

19 - Goddess Revolved Ankle Touches

Goal: Develop mobility through the shoulders, spine, and hips

Difficulty: ★★★★★

Description: In a Goddess Pose, add a revolved twist to reach and touch opposite ankles, combining a deep hip opener with a twisting motion for increased flexibility and core engagement.

Step-by-step:

1. Begin seated comfortably on the edge of your chair with your feet flat on the floor, placing them much wider than the hips, toes pointed outward in a goddess position.
2. Sit up tall, lengthening your spine, and engage your core muscles for stability.
3. Extend your arms out to the sides at shoulder height, palms facing forward.
4. Inhale deeply to prepare.
5. Exhale as you twist your torso to the right, bringing your left hand towards your right ankle or foot.
6. Keep your right arm extended out to the side, reaching towards the ceiling.
7. Engage your core muscles to support the twist and maintain stability.
8. Inhale to return to the center, bringing both arms back to shoulder height.
9. Exhale as you twist your torso to the left, bringing your right hand towards your left ankle or foot.
10. Keep your left arm extended out to the side, reaching towards the ceiling.
11. Engage your core muscles and maintain stability in the twist.
12. Inhale to return to the center and release the twist, bringing both arms back to shoulder height.
13. Repeat the sequence, flowing between the right and left twists, for 30–60 seconds.
14. Repeat 3–5 times.

Scan the QR code below for the video tutorial

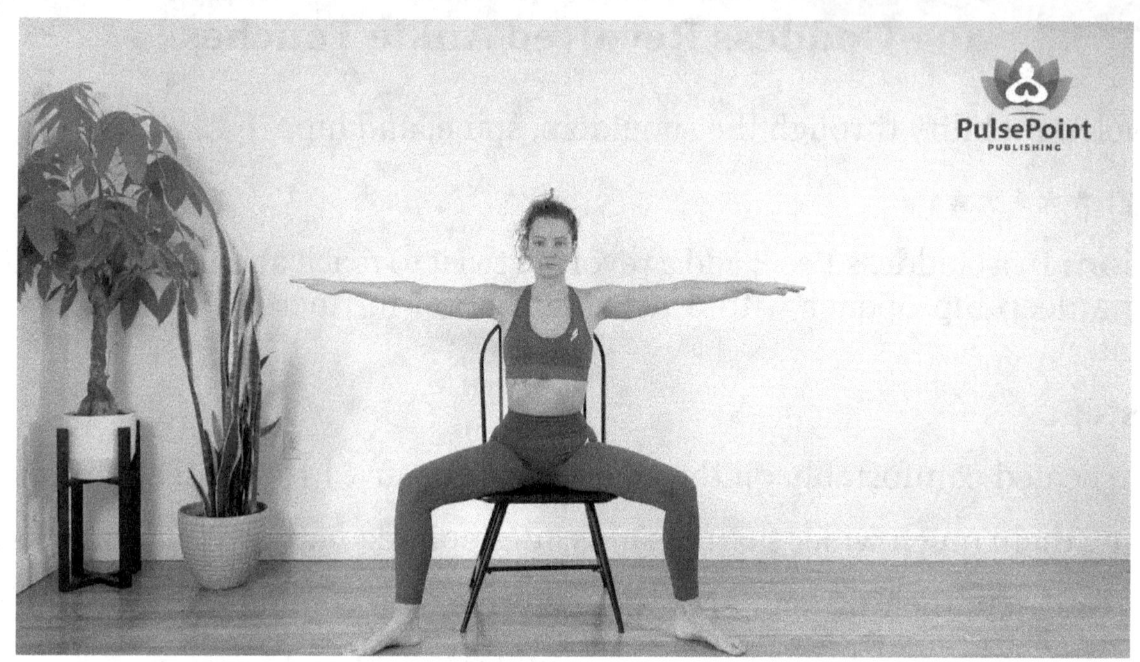

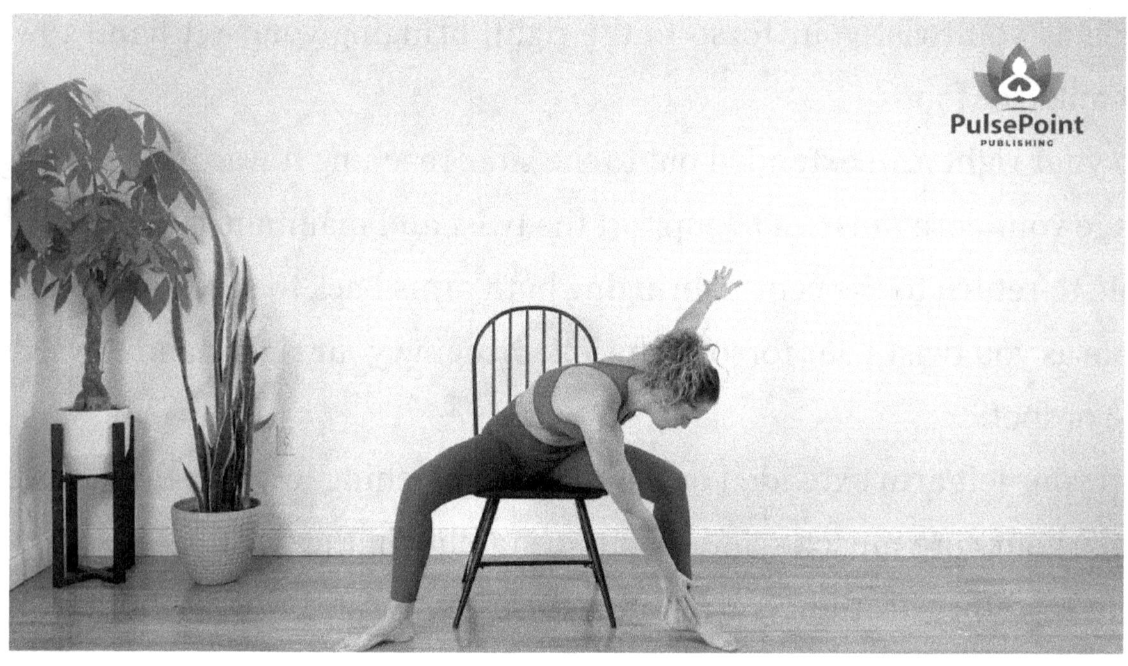

20 - Half Goddess Steps

Goal: Develop mobility through the hips

Difficulty: ★★★☆☆

Description: In a half Goddess Pose, take alternating steps side to side, engaging the lower body muscles to enhance mobility, endurance, and strengthen the inner thighs.

Step-by-step:

1. Begin seated comfortably on the edge of your chair with your feet flat on the floor, hip-width apart.
2. Sit up tall, lengthening your spine, and engage your core muscles for stability.
3. Begin to lift one foot off the floor and step it over to the side.
4. Lift that same foot off the floor and bring it back through the center.
5. Switch legs, stepping your food to the side and then back to center.
6. Repeat the sequence for 30–60 seconds.
7. Repeat 3–5 times.

Scan the QR code below for the video tutorial

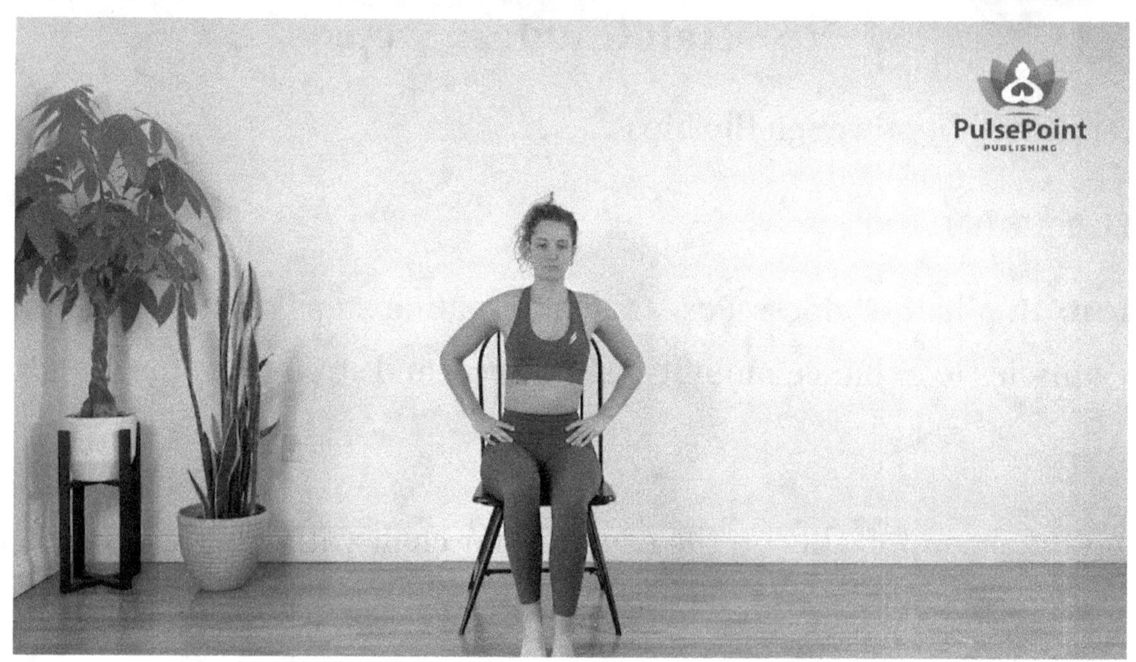

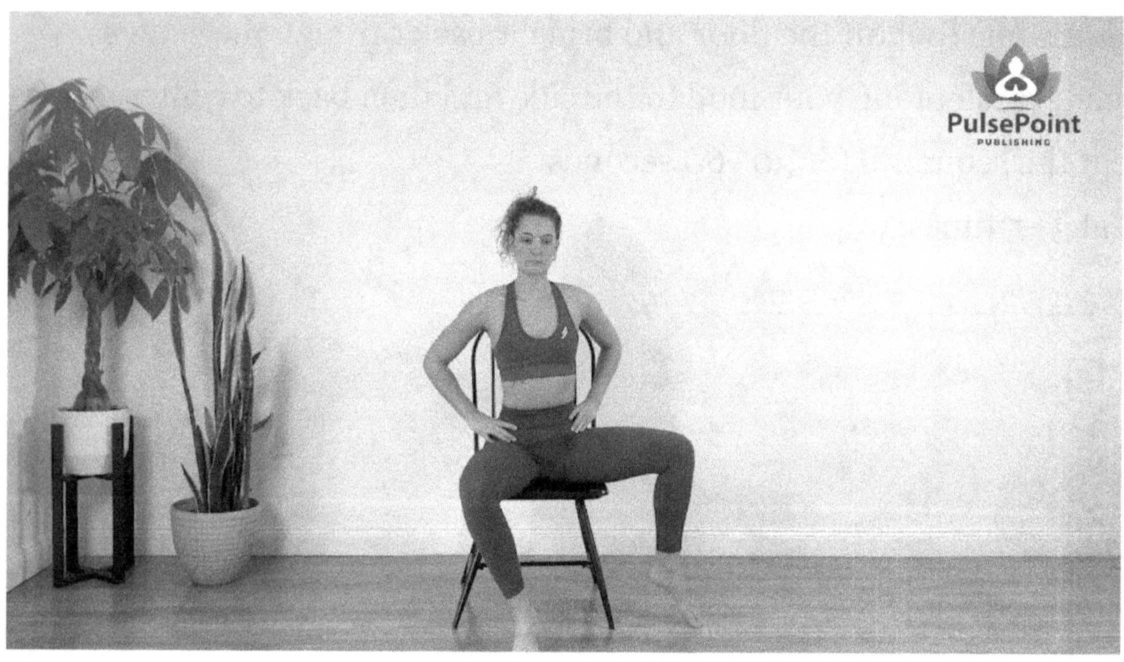

21 - Standing Lunge Twist

Goal: Increase the heart rate and develop mobility through the shoulders

Difficulty: ★★★★☆

Description: Finding dynamic movement in a standing lunch position but adding a twist through movement of the spine and arms.

Step-by-step:

1. Face the chair, standing with feet hips width apart.
2. Step one foot onto the chair, creating a 90-degree bend at the knee. Lean forward slightly onto the lifted foot.
3. Extend both arms up to the ceiling.
4. Keep your gaze forward, lengthen through your spine, and core engaged.
5. Inhale to reach up a little more.
6. Exhale, turn toward the side on your grounded leg. Drop your arms to the height of your shoulders.
7. Allow your gaze to follow your back hand.
8. Inhale, square your hips and shoulders back out, reaching your hands overhead.
9. Exhale to twist.
10. Continue through this movement for 30–60 seconds following your breath, and then switch sides.
11. Repeat 3–5 times.

Scan the QR code below for the video tutorial

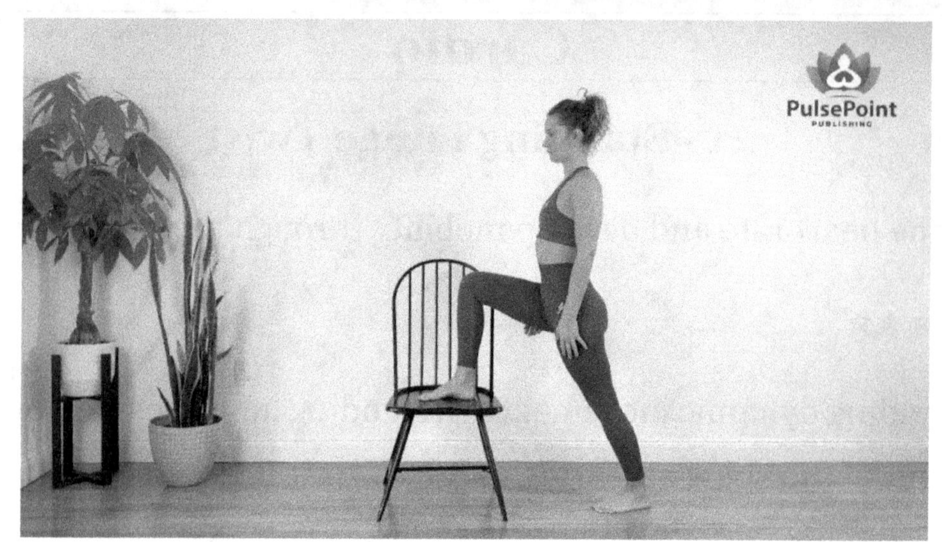

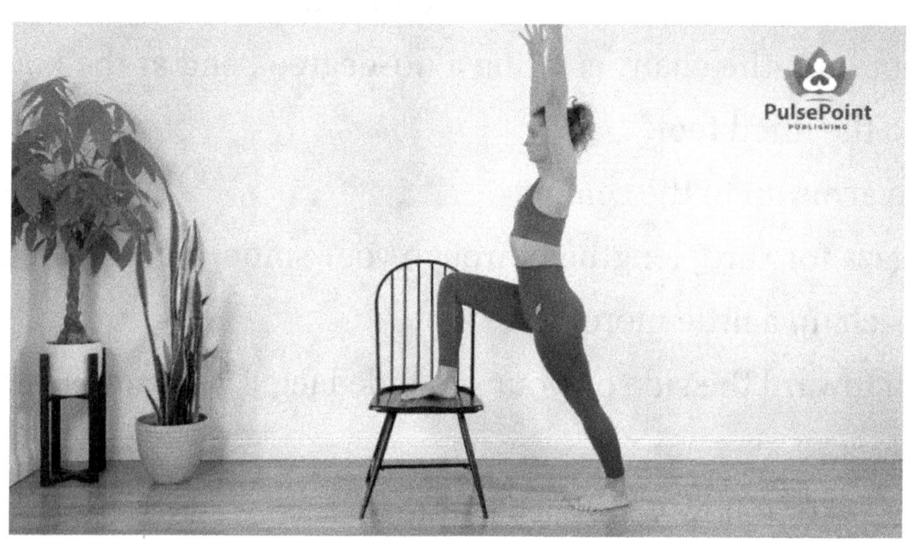

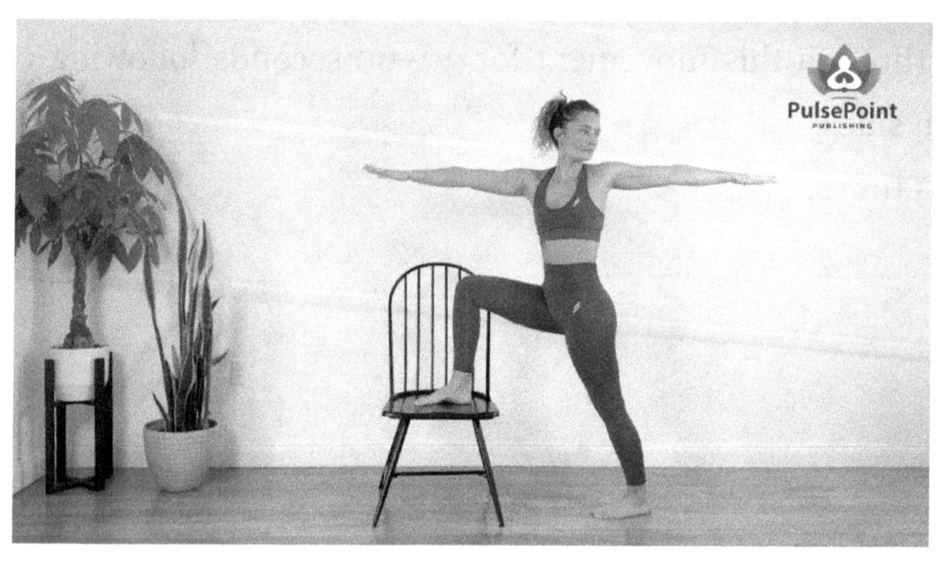

22 - Side Bend and Reach

Goal: Increase the heart rate and develop mobility through the shoulders and spine

Difficulty: ⅔

Description: In a seated side bend, adding a gentle twist and finding dynamic movement between the two.

Step-by-step:

1. Begin seated comfortably on the edge of your chair with your feet flat on the floor, hip-width apart.
2. Sit up tall, lengthening your spine, and place your hands on your thighs or the sides of the chair for support.
3. Inhale, reach your right arm overhead.
4. Exhale, fold over to your left side.
5. Keep your left hand grounded on your chair or thigh for support.
6. Use your core muscles to support your torso.
7. Keep both hips grounded on the chair and avoid leaning forward or backward.
8. Inhale to twist and reach your right arm further to the left, dropping your hand to the height of your shoulder.
9. Exhale, stack the shoulders back into the side bend.
10. Inhale, twist and reach.
11. Continue through this movement for 30–60 seconds, switching sides once complete.
12. Repeat 3–5 times.

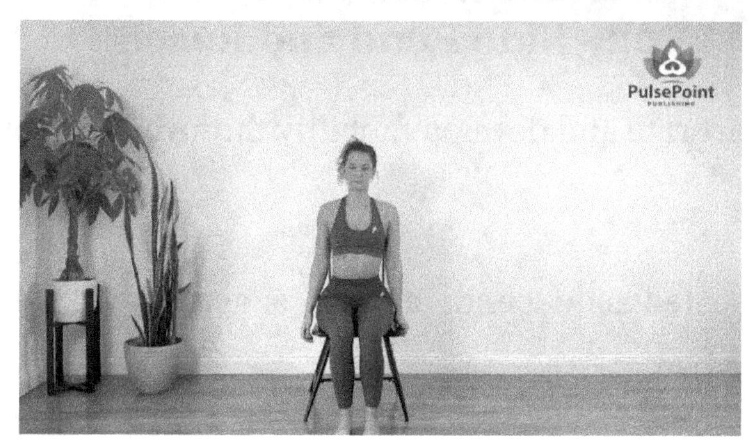

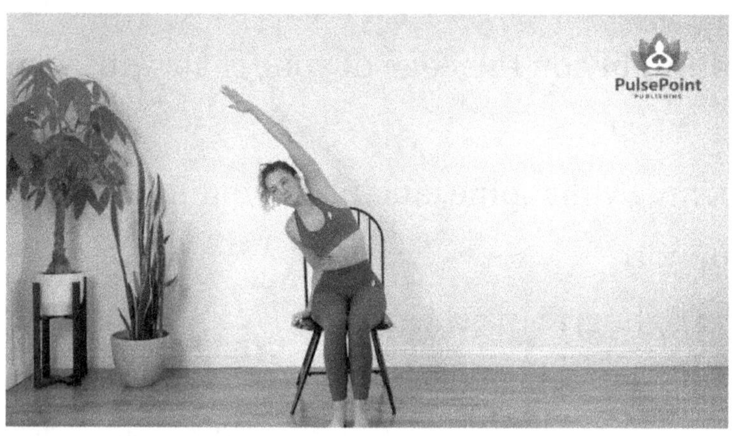

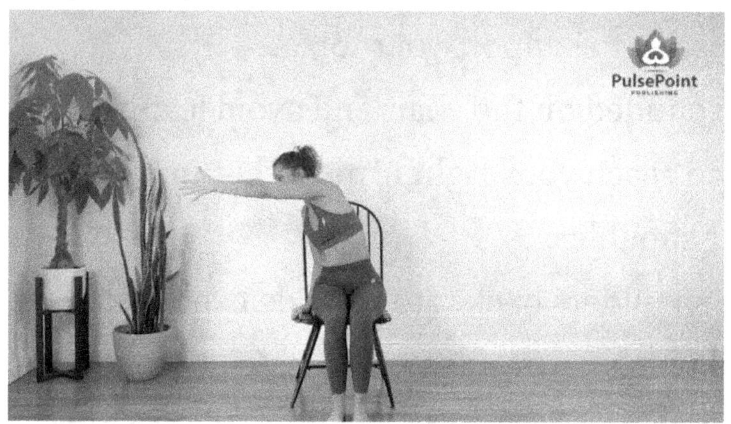

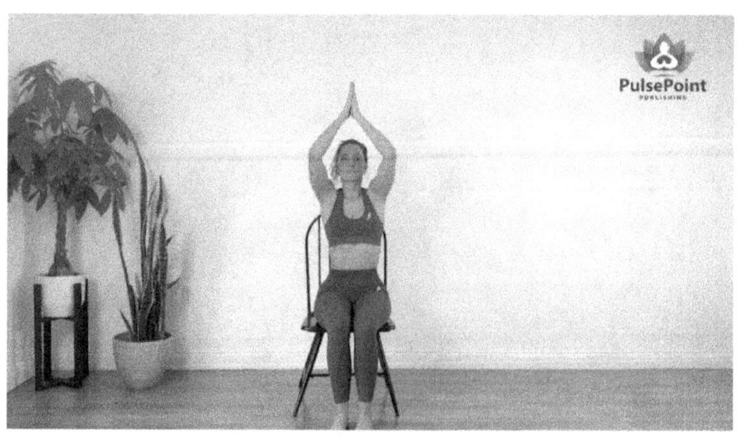

23 - Wide Legged Forward Fold Flow

Goal: Increase the heart rate and stretch the hips

Difficulty: ★★★☆☆

Description: Moving with breath, allowing the body to fall forward and upwards, creating dynamic movement between the two.

Step-by-step:

1. Begin seated comfortably on the edge of your chair with your feet flat on the floor, wider than hip-width apart.
2. Sit up tall, lengthening your spine, and engage your core muscles for stability.
3. Inhale, sweep your hands overhead, allow your gaze to follow if that's comfortable.
4. Exhale as you tilt at the hips and fold forward, placing your chest and arms between your legs.
5. Keep your spine long and extend your arms forward, reaching towards the floor.
6. Allow your head to hang heavy, relaxing your neck and shoulders.
7. Inhale to lift your torso all the way back up, reaching your hands overhead.
8. Exhale to fold back forward.
9. Continue through this flow for 30–60 seconds.
10. Repeat 3–5 times.

Scan the QR code below for the video tutorial

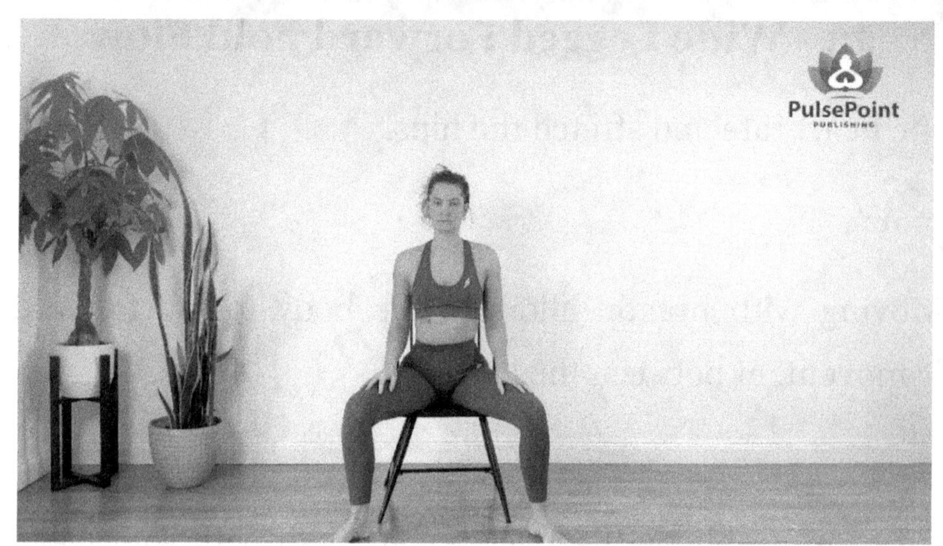

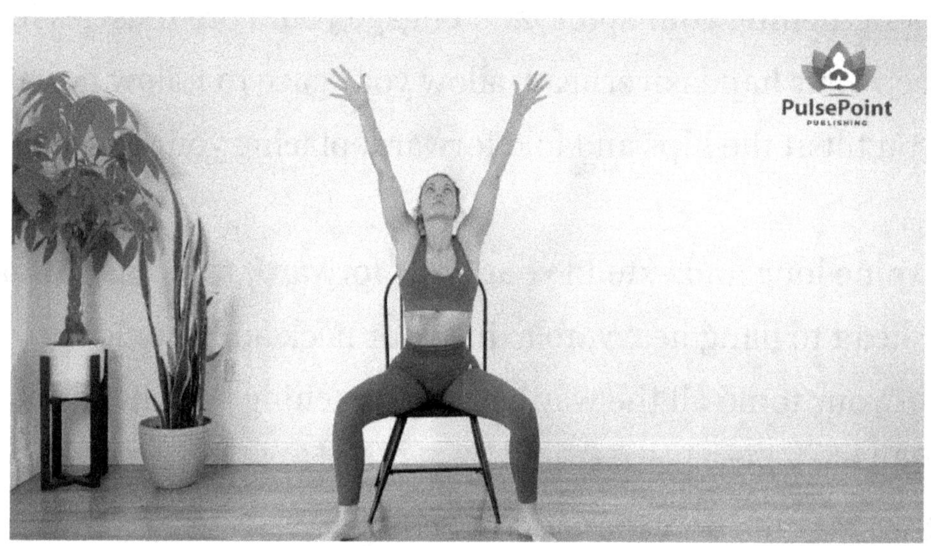

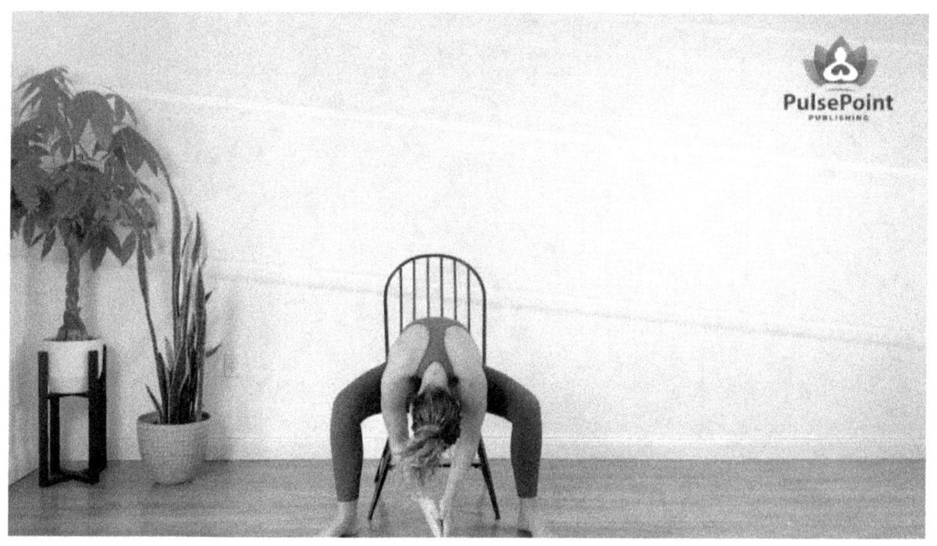

24 - Reverse Warrior Flow

Goal: Increase the heart rate and stretch the lats

Difficulty: ★★★★★

Description: From a Warrior II position, seamlessly moving into Reverse Warrior and back again, continuing movement between the two.

Step-by-step:

1. Begin seated comfortably on the edge of your chair with your feet flat on the floor, hip-width apart.
2. Sit up tall, lengthening your spine, and engage your core muscles for stability.
3. Extend your arms out to the sides at shoulder height, palms facing down, coming into a wide-legged stance.
4. Turn your right foot out to the right, so the toes point towards the side of the chair.
5. Keep your left foot pointing forward or slightly turned inwards.
6. Bend your right knee, bringing it directly over your right ankle, coming into a modified Warrior II position.
7. Ensure your right knee is in line with your right ankle, and your thigh is parallel to the floor.
8. Keep your left leg straight and strong, pressing firmly into the floor.
9. Gaze over your right fingertips, extending your vision beyond your right hand.
10. Engage your core muscles to support your torso and maintain stability.
11. Inhale, flip your front palm up to the ceiling.
12. Exhale, reverse your warrior. Send your left arm down your back leg, and your right up upwards. The gaze can follow your lifted arm.
13. Inhale lift back to center.
14. Exhale, reverse your warrior.
15. Continue through this movement for 30–60 seconds, and switch sides.
16. Repeat each side 3–5 times.

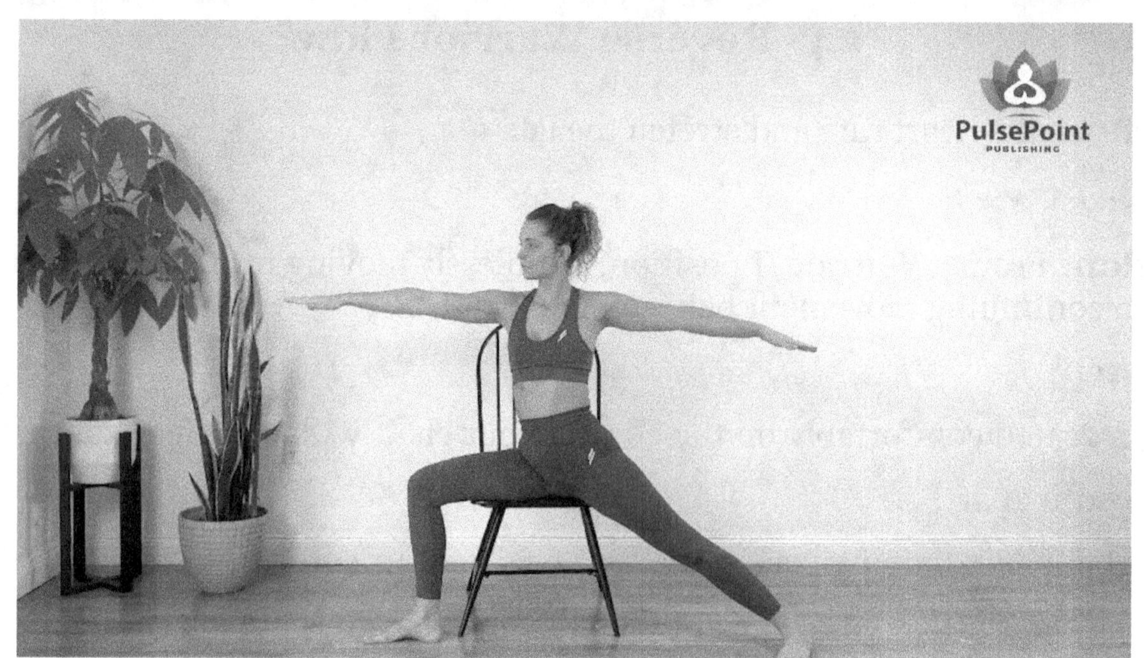

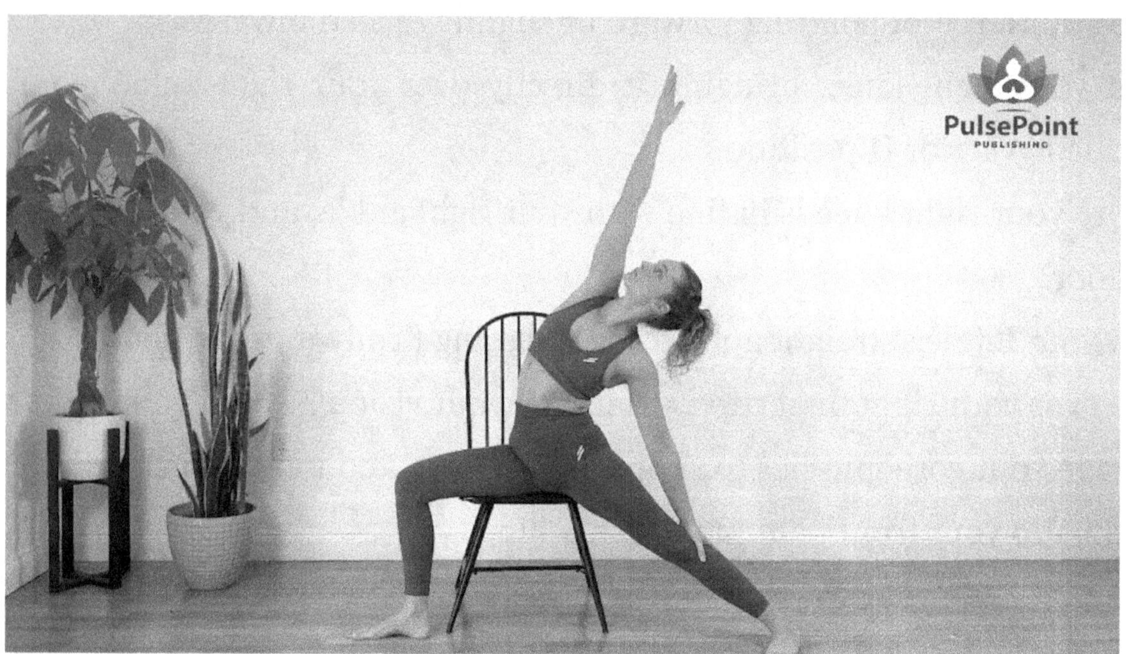

25 - Warrior II Arm Extensions

Goal: Increase the heart rate and strengthen the lower body
Difficulty: ★★★☆☆
Description: From a Warrior II position, adding in dynamic arm movements.
Step-by-step:

1. Begin seated comfortably on the edge of your chair with your feet flat on the floor, hip-width apart.
2. Sit up tall, lengthening your spine, and engage your core muscles for stability.
3. Extend your arms out to the sides at shoulder height, palms facing down, coming into a wide-legged stance.
4. Turn your right foot out to the right, so the toes point towards the side of the chair.
5. Keep your left foot pointing forward or slightly turned inwards.
6. Bend your right knee, bringing it directly over your right ankle, coming into a modified Warrior II position.
7. Ensure your right knee is in line with your right ankle, and your thigh is parallel to the floor.
8. Keep your left leg straight and strong, pressing firmly into the floor.
9. Gaze over your right fingertips, extending your vision beyond your right hand.
10. Engage your core muscles to support your torso and maintain stability.
11. Inhale, reach your arms a little further.
12. Exhale, draw your elbows in towards your body bringing your shoulder blades together.
13. Inhale, reach the arms back out.
14. Continue this movement with your breath for 30–60 seconds, making sure to switch sides once complete.
15. Repeat each side 3–5 times.

Scan the QR code for the video tutorial

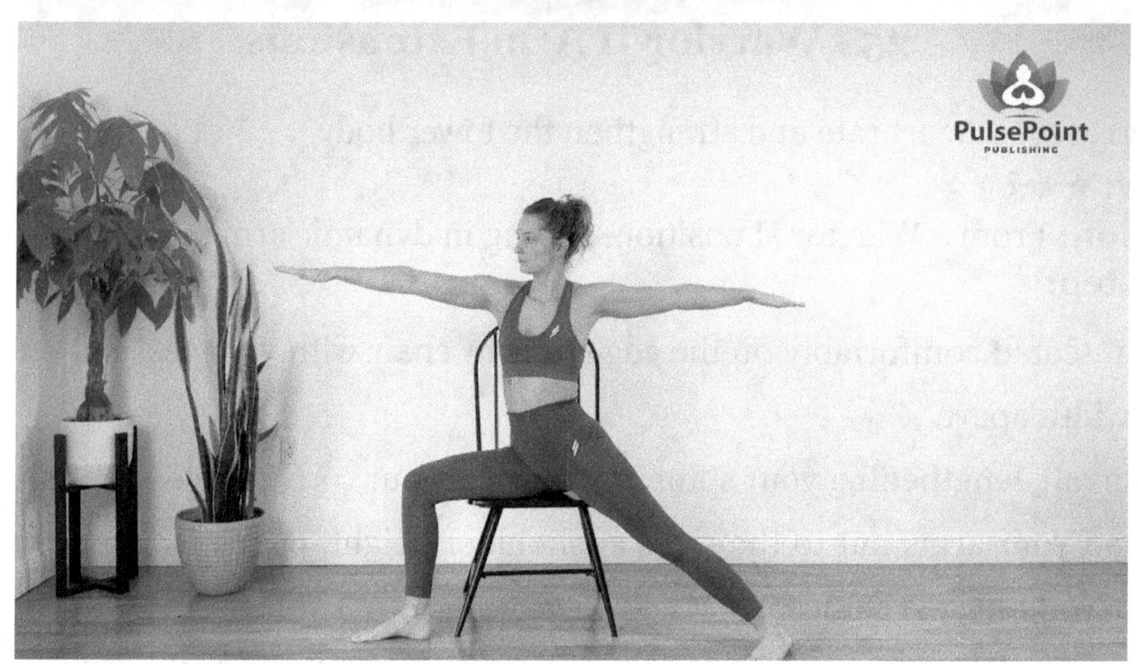

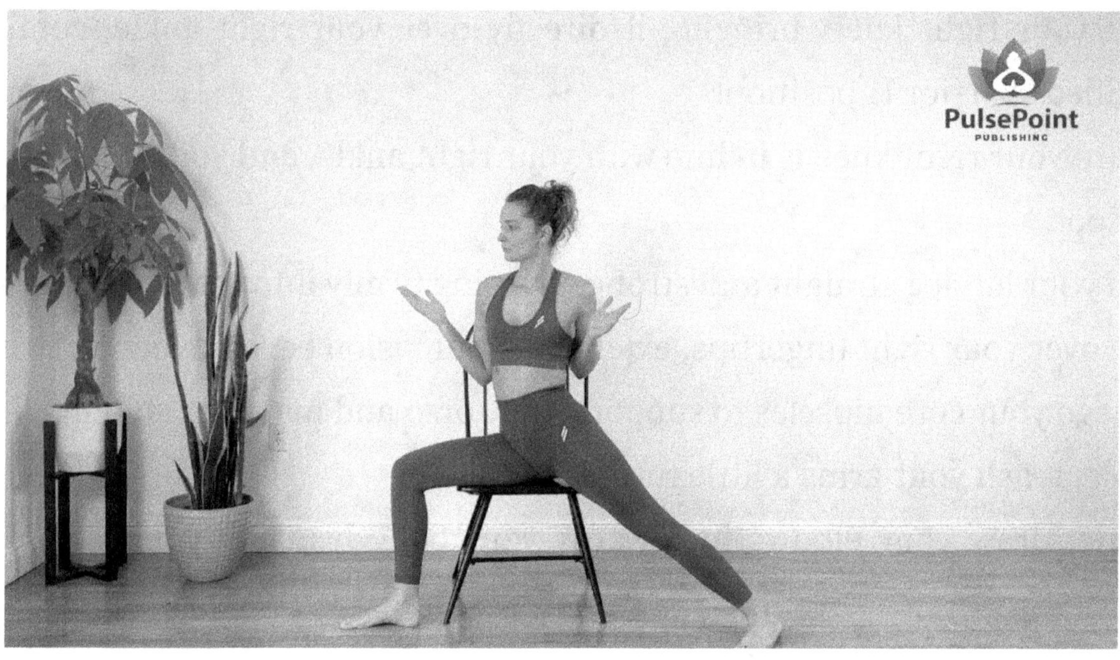

CHAPTER 5: COMPREHENSIVE WELL-BEING WITH CHAIR YOGA

One of the key benefits of chair yoga is its ability to improve flexibility, strength, and balance. Through gentle movements and stretches, participants can gradually increase their range of motion and develop a stronger core. These physical benefits contribute to overall well-being and can help prevent injuries and improve posture.

In addition to the physical benefits, chair yoga improves mental and emotional wellbeing. The practice promotes mindfulness, which is being completely present in the moment and paying attention to one's thoughts and feelings without passing judgment. Chair yoga, which incorporates breathing techniques and meditation, helps to relieve tension and anxiety while also fostering peace and relaxation.

What makes chair yoga particularly appealing is its accessibility. It is a gentle form of yoga that can be adapted to suit individuals of all ages and abilities. Whether you are a beginner or have limited mobility, chair yoga offers modifications and variations that allow everyone to participate and experience the benefits.

Yoga for Holistic Health

Chair yoga is a practice that offers a comprehensive approach to enhancing physical, mental, and emotional health. Through a series of gentle and modified yoga poses, chair yoga provides numerous benefits that contribute to overall well-being.

One of the primary advantages of chair yoga is its ability to improve flexibility, strength, and balance. The practice involves gentle stretching and movement of the body, which helps to increase flexibility and range of motion. This is particularly beneficial for individuals with limited mobility or those recovering from injuries. By strengthening the muscles, chair yoga also enhances stability and balance, reducing the risk of falls and injuries.

In addition to the physical benefits, chair yoga has a profound impact on mental and emotional health. The practice promotes mindfulness, which is being completely present in the moment and developing a nonjudgmental awareness of one's thoughts and experiences. By focusing on the breath and the body's movements, chair yoga promotes a sense of calm and relaxation, reducing stress and anxiety. Regular practice can also improve mental clarity, concentration, and overall emotional well-being.

Chair yoga is accessible to individuals of all ages and abilities, making it a suitable practice for everyone. The use of a chair provides support and stability, allowing individuals with physical limitations or disabilities to participate fully. The practice can be adapted to meet individual needs, ensuring a safe and comfortable experience for all. Whether young or old, fit or sedentary, chair yoga offers a gentle yet effective way to improve overall health and well-being.

In all, chair yoga is a holistic approach to health that encompasses physical, mental, and emotional well-being. Chair yoga, which uses moderate movements and mindfulness, increases flexibility, strength, and balance while lowering stress and encouraging relaxation.

Its accessibility makes it an ideal practice for individuals of all ages and abilities. Embrace the comprehensive benefits of chair yoga and embark on a journey towards holistic health.

Emotional and Spiritual Wellness

Chair yoga is not only beneficial for physical health but also plays a significant role in supporting emotional and spiritual well-being. The practice of chair yoga emphasizes the connection between physical movement and the enhancement of emotional and spiritual wellness.

One of the key benefits of chair yoga for emotional well-being is stress reduction. The gentle and modified yoga poses help release tension and promote relaxation, allowing individuals to let go of stress and anxiety. The slow and controlled movements in chair yoga encourage deep breathing, which activates the body's relaxation response and calms the nervous system. This can have a profound impact on emotional well-being by reducing feelings of overwhelm and promoting a sense of inner peace.

Chair yoga also promotes mindfulness, which is an essential aspect of emotional and spiritual wellness. Mindfulness entails being completely present in the moment while nonjudgmentally examining one's thoughts, feelings, and experiences. Through chair yoga, individuals are encouraged to focus their attention on the sensations of the body, the breath, and the present moment. This cultivates a state of mindfulness, allowing individuals to develop a greater sense of self-awareness and a deeper connection with their inner selves.

In addition to stress reduction and mindfulness, chair yoga provides opportunities for relaxation and self-care. The practice includes gentle stretching and relaxation exercises that help release physical and mental tension. These relaxation techniques can be particularly beneficial for individuals who are experiencing emotional distress or struggling with mental health issues. Chair yoga offers a safe and supportive environment for individuals to take time for themselves, nurture their bodies, and cultivate a sense of inner calm.

Specific techniques and poses in chair yoga can be practiced to promote emotional and spiritual well-being. For example, deep breathing exercises, such as diaphragmatic breathing or alternate nostril breathing, can help regulate emotions and promote a sense of calm. Gentle twists and forward bends can release tension in the spine and promote a sense of grounding. Heart-opening poses, such as the seated cat-cow stretch or the seated spinal twist, can help individuals connect with their emotions and open their hearts to self-compassion and acceptance.

Overall, chair yoga offers a holistic approach to enhancing emotional and spiritual well-being. By incorporating gentle movement, mindfulness, relaxation, and self-awareness, chair yoga supports individuals in their journey towards emotional balance, inner peace, and a deeper connection with their spiritual selves.

CHAPTER 6: EXPANDING YOUR CHAIR YOGA JOURNEY

As you continue your chair yoga practice, you may find yourself eager to explore new horizons and delve deeper into the world of this gentle yet powerful form of exercise. Introducing advanced poses, modifications, and variations, and incorporating mindfulness and breathing techniques into sessions can expand your chair yoga journey.

1. Advanced Chair Yoga Poses

Once you have mastered the foundational chair yoga poses, it's time to challenge yourself with more advanced variations. These poses will strengthen your body while also improving your mind-body connection. Here are some samples to help you get started:

a. Eagle Arms Twist: Sit tall in your chair, cross your right arm over your left arm, and intertwine your forearms. Inhale deeply, then exhale as you twist your torso to the right, hooking your left elbow outside your right knee. Hold the pose for a few breaths, feeling the stretch in your upper back and shoulders. Repeat on the other side.

b. Warrior II Chair Pose: Begin by sitting on the edge of your chair with your feet hip-width apart. Extend your right leg straight out in front of you while bending your left knee, creating a 90-degree angle. Raise your arms parallel to the floor, with your right arm reaching forward and your left arm reaching backward. Hold the pose for several breaths, feeling the strength and stability in your legs and core. Repeat on the other side.

2. Modifications and Variations

Chair yoga is a practice that can be adapted to suit individuals of all abilities and physical conditions. If you have specific limitations or injuries, it's important to modify poses to ensure your safety and comfort. Here are some changes and alterations to consider:

a. Seated Cat-Cow: While seated in your chair, place your hands on your thighs. Inhale deeply, arching your spine and lifting your chest (Cow Pose). Exhale as you round your back, tucking your chin towards your chest (Cat Pose). Repeat this gentle movement, synchronizing it with your breath, to release tension in your spine.

b. Seated Pigeon Pose: Sit towards the edge of your chair and cross your right ankle over your left thigh. Flex your right foot to protect your knee. Gently push down on your right knee to increase the stretch in your hip. Hold for a few breaths and then swap sides.

3. Mindfulness and Breathing Techniques

Chair yoga is not just about physical movement; it is also an opportunity to cultivate mindfulness and connect with your breath. Incorporating these strategies into your practice can aid in relaxation, stress reduction, and general well-being. Here are some ways to try:

a. Mindful Breathing: Sit comfortably in your chair, close your eyes, and bring your attention to your breath. Take calm, deep breaths, concentrating on the sensation of the air entering and exiting your body. Allow any ideas or distractions to pass without judgment, then restore your concentration to your breathing.

b. Body Scan Meditation: Begin at the top of your head and gradually move your focus to each region of your body, noting any feelings or places of stress. As you breathe, imagine sending your breath to those areas, allowing them to relax and release any tension. Move down through your body, scanning and relaxing each part, until you reach your toes.

4. Additional Resources

To further enrich your chair yoga journey, we recommend exploring additional resources such as books, videos, and workshops. These resources can provide you with valuable insights, inspiration, and guidance. Here are a few suggestions:

• Chair Yoga: Sit, Stretch, and Strengthen Your Way to a Happier, Healthier You by Kristin McGee

• Gentle Chair Yoga: A Comprehensive Guide to Daily Practice by James F. Winters

• Online videos and tutorials by renowned chair yoga instructors such as Lakshmi Voelker and Peggy Cappy

• Local workshops or classes offered by yoga studios or community centers.

Advanced Concepts in Chair Yoga

The execution of advanced chair yoga poses is vital for reaping the benefits of the actions Learning how to safely perform challenging poses while seated on a chair, with clear and detailed instructions will provide the information to progress in one's practice. Modifications and variations of these poses will also, allow individuals of different abilities to adapt the practice to their needs.

In addition to the physical aspects, the importance of incorporating mindfulness and breathing techniques into chair yoga sessions help cultivate a sense of relaxation and heightened awareness through the integration of these practices. The benefits of mindfulness and conscious breathing include positive effects on mental and emotional well-being.

Furthermore, the applications of advanced chair yoga for different populations and specific health conditions can be used therapeutically to improve strength, flexibility, balance, and overall well-being.

To support individuals in their exploration of advanced chair yoga, investigating additional resources such as books, videos, and workshops. will enable individuals to further deepen their knowledge and expand their practice.

By incorporating these advanced techniques, individuals can continue to reap the numerous physical, mental, and emotional benefits that chair yoga has to offer.

Beyond the Chair

Yoga is often associated with serene studio settings and practitioners contorting their bodies into various poses on mats. However, the practice of yoga extends far beyond the boundaries of the traditional yoga mat, reaching into the realms of lifestyle and community involvement.

While traditional yoga poses are typically performed on the ground, chair yoga offers a unique approach that caters to individuals with limited mobility or those who prefer a seated practice. Advanced chair yoga poses provide a gentle yet effective workout, targeting muscles, improving flexibility, and enhancing overall well-being. By incorporating modifications and adaptations, chair yoga can be customized to suit a wide range of abilities and needs.

But chair yoga is not just about physical movement; it encompasses a holistic approach to wellness. Mindfulness, a central tenet of yoga, plays a significant role in chair yoga practice. By cultivating present-moment awareness, individuals can tap into a deeper connection with their bodies, thoughts, and emotions. This heightened self-awareness fosters a sense of calm, reduces stress, and promotes mental clarity.

Conscious breathing techniques further enhance the benefits of chair yoga. By focusing on the breath, practitioners can regulate their nervous system, inducing relaxation and tranquility. Deep, intentional breaths oxygenate the body, invigorating the mind and promoting a sense of vitality. The controlled breathwork in chair yoga not only improves lung capacity but also cultivates a peaceful state of mind.

The implications of chair yoga extend beyond individual well-being, extending into the realm of community involvement. Chair yoga classes provide a safe and inclusive space for individuals of all ages, abilities, and backgrounds to come together and share a transformative experience. The practice fosters a sense of belonging and connection, breaking down barriers and promoting social cohesion.

Moreover, chair yoga can be tailored to meet the specific needs of different populations and health conditions. From seniors seeking to improve balance and mobility to individuals with chronic pain or disabilities, chair yoga offers a gentle yet effective way to enhance physical and mental health. By adapting the practice to address specific concerns and limitations, chair yoga becomes a powerful tool for promoting overall well-being and inclusivity.

For those interested in delving deeper into the world of chair yoga, there is a wealth of resources available. Books, online courses, and instructional videos provide comprehensive guidance and support for both practitioners and instructors. By expanding our knowledge and understanding of chair yoga, we can further harness its potential to positively impact individuals and communities.

In all, the broader implications of yoga on lifestyle and community involvement extend far beyond the confines of a yoga mat. Chair yoga, with its advanced poses, modifications, mindfulness practices, and conscious breathing techniques, offers a unique approach to wellness that caters to diverse populations. By embracing chair yoga, individuals can improve their physical and mental well-being, while fostering a sense of community and inclusivity. Let us embark on this transformative journey, exploring the boundless possibilities that lie beyond the chair.

Glossary of Terms

Welcome to our comprehensive glossary of common yoga terms. This guide aims to provide you with a thorough understanding of the various terms and concepts used in yoga. Whether you're a beginner or an experienced practitioner, this glossary will serve as a valuable reference tool to enhance your understanding and practice of yoga.

1. Asana: Asana refers to the physical postures and poses practiced in yoga. These postures are designed to promote strength, flexibility, and balance, while also cultivating mindfulness and focus.

2. Pranayama: Pranayama is the practice of breath control in yoga. It involves various techniques to regulate and manipulate the breath, which can have a profound impact on our physical, mental, and emotional well-being.

3. Meditation: Meditation is a practice that involves training the mind to achieve a state of deep relaxation and heightened awareness. It cultivates mindfulness, clarity, and inner peace, allowing us to connect with our true selves.

4. Om: Om is a sacred sound and a spiritual symbol in yoga. It represents the universal consciousness and serves as a mantra to focus the mind during meditation and chanting.

5. Chakra: Chakras are energy centers located along the spine. There are seven primary chakras, each representing a particular quality or facet of our existence. Balancing and activating these chakras can promote physical, emotional, and spiritual well-being.

6. Namaste: Namaste is a common greeting in yoga, often accompanied by a gesture of placing the palms together at the heart center. It is a way of acknowledging the divine spark within ourselves and others, and a gesture of respect and gratitude.

7. Savasana: Savasana, also known as Corpse Pose, is a relaxation posture practiced at the end of a yoga session. It involves lying flat on the back, completely surrendering the body and mind, allowing for deep relaxation and integration of the practice.

8. Vinyasa: Vinyasa refers to a flowing sequence of yoga poses that are synchronized with the breath. It is a dynamic and energetic style of yoga that builds strength, flexibility, and endurance.

9. Hatha: Hatha yoga is a branch of yoga that focuses on physical postures (asanas) and breath control (pranayama). It aims to balance the opposing energies within us, creating harmony between the body and mind.

10. Mudra: Mudras are hand gestures used in yoga and meditation to channel and direct energy. Each mudra has a specific meaning and purpose, and when practiced with intention, can enhance the overall yoga experience.

11. Ujjayi: Ujjayi breath is a specific breathing technique used in yoga. Constricting the back of the neck while inhaling produces a quiet hissing sound. Ujjayi breath regulates the breath, improves attention, and generates interior heat.

12. Dhyana: Dhyana, or contemplation, is a state of deep meditation where the mind is completely absorbed and focused. It is a practice of observing thoughts without attachment or judgment, allowing for greater clarity and insight.

This glossary provides just a glimpse into the vast world of yoga terminology. By familiarizing yourself with these terms and their meanings, you'll be well-equipped to navigate the yoga practice with confidence and understanding. Whether you're attending a yoga class, reading a book, or exploring online resources, this glossary will be your trusted companion on your yoga journey.

Remember, yoga is not only about the physical exercise; it is a comprehensive approach to well-being that includes the body, mind, and spirit. So, dive in, explore, and embrace the transformative power of yoga. Namaste!

Recommended Resources

In the world of chair yoga, there is a wealth of resources available to help you dive deeper into this gentle yet powerful practice. Whether you're a beginner looking to learn the basics or an experienced practitioner seeking to expand your knowledge, the following comprehensive list of resources will guide you on your journey towards a healthier mind and body.

1. Books

• Chair Yoga: Sit, Stretch, and Strengthen Your Way to a Happier, Healthier You by Kristin McGee: This book serves as an excellent introduction to chair yoga, offering clear and concise instructions on various poses and sequences. It also provides insights into the benefits of chair yoga and how it can be integrated into daily life.

• Yoga for Seniors: Chair Yoga for All Ages by Lynn Lehmkuhl: Specifically tailored for seniors, this book offers a gentle approach to chair yoga, focusing on improving flexibility, balance, and overall well-being. It includes detailed explanations of each pose, accompanied by helpful illustrations.

• The Complete Guide to Chair Yoga: The Definitive Resource for Teachers and Students by Eyal Shifroni: This comprehensive guide is a must-have for both yoga teachers and students. It covers a wide range of chair yoga techniques, modifications, and adaptations for different populations, making it a valuable resource for those looking to deepen their understanding of the practice.

2. Websites

• Yoga Journal (www.yogajournal.com): This popular website features a dedicated section on chair yoga, offering articles, videos, and tutorials for practitioners of all levels. It provides a wealth of information on various chair yoga poses, their benefits, and modifications.

• Yoga International (www.yogainternational.com): With its extensive library of online classes and articles, Yoga International is a valuable resource for chair yoga enthusiasts. The website offers specialized chair yoga classes, workshops, and expert advice to help you refine your practice.

• SilverSneakers (www.silversneakers.com): Designed for older adults, SilverSneakers provides a range of fitness programs, including chair yoga. Their website offers a collection of chair yoga videos led by experienced instructors, allowing you to practice from the comfort of your own home.

3. Other Resources

• YouTube: A treasure trove of chair yoga videos, YouTube offers a vast array of tutorials, guided practices, and full-length classes. From gentle stretches to more challenging sequences, you can find a variety of chair yoga resources to suit your needs and preferences.

• Local Community Centers: Many community centers offer chair yoga classes as part of their wellness programs. These classes provide an opportunity to practice in a supportive and inclusive environment, guided by experienced instructors who can offer personalized guidance and modifications.

• Social Media Groups: Joining chair yoga communities on platforms like Facebook and Instagram can connect you with like-minded individuals who share their experiences, insights, and resources. These groups often provide a platform for discussions, Q&A sessions, and even live-streamed classes.

While the resources mentioned above cover a wide range of chair yoga materials, it is important to note that this list is not exhaustive. There are numerous other books, websites, and resources available that can further enhance your understanding and practice of chair yoga.

Remember, the journey of chair yoga is a personal one, and it's essential to find resources that resonate with you and support your individual needs. Explore these recommended resources, and let them guide you towards a deeper appreciation of the transformative power of chair yoga.

CHAPTER 8: CONCLUSION

Throughout the chapters, we have discussed various chair yoga poses and their benefits. These poses are specifically designed to be accessible for individuals with varied educational backgrounds, including those with high school to college education.

One of the key themes that emerged from our discussions is the importance of incorporating movement into our daily lives, regardless of age or physical ability. Chair yoga provides a gentle yet effective way to stay active and improve flexibility, strength, and balance.

We have also emphasized the importance of mindfulness and breath awareness in chair yoga. By focusing on our breath and being present in the moment, we can cultivate a sense of calm and relaxation. This can be particularly beneficial for individuals with stressful lifestyles or those looking to manage anxiety and improve mental well-being.

Another theme that has been highlighted is the adaptability of chair yoga. Whether you are at home, in the office, or traveling, you can easily incorporate chair yoga into your routine. The use of a chair as a prop allows for modifications and variations of poses, making it accessible to individuals with different physical abilities.

Furthermore, we have discussed the potential health benefits of chair yoga, such as improved circulation, reduced joint pain, and increased energy levels. These benefits make chair yoga a valuable practice for individuals of all ages and backgrounds.

Reflecting on the Journey

The transformative power and benefits of chair yoga for seniors have been discussed throughout this book. We have explored the numerous ways in which chair yoga has positively impacted the physical, mental, and emotional well-being of seniors.

One of the primary advantages of chair yoga is the potential to increase flexibility, strength, and balance. Seniors who practiced modest stretching and mobility activities reported higher joint range of motion, increased muscular strength, and better overall balance. These physical improvements not only contribute to a better quality of life but also help prevent falls and injuries.

In addition to the physical benefits, chair yoga has proven to be a valuable tool in reducing stress and promoting relaxation. The combination of mindful movement and breath awareness has allowed seniors to release tension, calm their minds, and find inner peace. This practice of mindfulness has been particularly beneficial in managing anxiety and improving overall mental well-being.

Furthermore, chair yoga has provided seniors with a sense of community and connection. By participating in group classes or practicing with others, seniors have found a supportive and inclusive environment where they can share their experiences and build relationships. This sense of belonging has helped to overcome the loneliness and isolation that many elders experience.

As we conclude this journey, it is important to emphasize the holistic nature of chair yoga. It is more than simply physical exercise; it is a discipline that benefits the body, mind, and soul.

Chair yoga offers a safe and accessible form of exercise for seniors, regardless of their fitness level or mobility limitations. It empowers them to take control of their health and well-being, promoting a greater sense of independence and vitality.

Incorporating chair yoga into daily life can truly be life-changing for seniors. It has the potential to enhance their physical capabilities, reduce stress, foster a sense of community, and promote overall health and well-being. As we reflect on this journey, let us continue to embrace and explore the transformative power of chair yoga, ensuring a happier and healthier future for ourselves and our loved ones.

Looking Forward

In today's fast-paced world, where stress and sedentary lifestyles have become the norm, it is essential to find ways to prioritize our physical, mental, and social well-being. Chair yoga offers a unique and accessible approach to holistic wellness, allowing individuals of all ages and abilities to reap the benefits of yoga without the need for a mat or complicated poses. By encouraging ongoing practice and exploration in the realm of chair yoga, we can unlock a multitude of benefits that enhance our overall quality of life.

Physical Benefits

Chair yoga provides a gentle yet effective way to improve flexibility, strength, and balance. The practice incorporates modified yoga poses that are adapted to be performed while seated or supported by a chair. These poses help to increase joint mobility, enhance blood circulation, and promote better posture. By engaging in regular chair yoga sessions, individuals can experience improved muscle tone, reduced stiffness, and increased energy levels. The practice also aids in relieving chronic pain and tension, making it an excellent option for those with physical limitations or mobility issues.

Mental Benefits

The mind-body connection is a fundamental aspect of chair yoga, and it offers numerous mental health benefits. By focusing on breath control and mindful movement, chair yoga cultivates a sense of inner calm, reducing stress and anxiety levels. The practice encourages individuals to be fully present in the moment, fostering a state of mindfulness that can be carried into everyday life. Regular chair yoga practice has been shown to improve cognitive function, memory, and concentration. It also provides an opportunity for self-reflection and introspection, promoting a positive mindset and emotional well-being.

Social Benefits

Chair yoga is not just an individual practice; it can also be a fantastic way to build connections and foster a sense of community. Group chair yoga classes create a supportive and inclusive environment where individuals can come together, share their experiences, and support one another on their wellness journeys. The practice encourages social interaction, boosting self-confidence and reducing feelings of isolation. Chair yoga classes often incorporate partner poses and group activities, promoting teamwork and camaraderie. By engaging in chair yoga as a social activity, individuals can forge new friendships and strengthen existing relationships.

In conclusion, chair yoga offers a holistic approach to well-being, encompassing physical, mental, and social benefits. By encouraging ongoing practice and exploration in the realm of chair yoga, individuals can experience improved flexibility, strength, balance, reduced stress, enhanced cognitive function, and a sense of belonging within a supportive community. So, grab a chair, take a seat, and embark on a journey towards holistic well-being through the practice of chair yoga.

CHAPTER 9: 28 DAY CHAIR YOGA CHALLENGE

Day 1: Stretch & Strength	Day 2: Balance & Cardio

- Low lunge backbend
  - Hold for 45 seconds
  - Release for 30 seconds
  - Repeat 3 times
- Chair pose flow
  - Move for 60 seconds
  - Take a 30 second break
  - Repeat 5 times
- Seated forward fold
  - Hold for 60 seconds
  - Take a 30 second break
  - Repeat 4 times
- Goddess side crunches
  - Move for 45 seconds
  - Take a 45 second break
  - Repeat 3 times

- Palm tree
  - Hold for 60 seconds
  - Repeat on the other leg
  - Take a 30 second break
  - Repeat each side 3 times
- Wide legged forward fold flow
  - Move for 45 seconds
  - Take a 30 second break
  - Repeat 5 times
- Standing lunge twist
  - Move for 45 seconds
  - Repeat on the other side
  - Take a 30 second break
  - Repeat each side 4 times
- Warrior II arm extension
  - Move for 60 seconds
  - Repeat on the other side
  - Take a 30 second break
  - Repeat each side 3 times

<table>
<tr><td>

Day 3: Mobility & Stretch

- Triangle pose arm rotations
  - Move for 30 seconds
  - Repeat on the other side
  - Take a 45 second break
  - Repeat each side 2 times
- Seated twist
  - Hold for 30 seconds
  - Repeat on the other side
  - Take a 30 second break
  - Repeat each side 3 times
- Seated pigeon
  - Hold for 60 seconds
  - Repeat on the other side
  - Take a 30 second break
  - Repeat on each side 4 times
- Overhead shoulder stretch
  - Hold for 30 seconds
  - Take a 30 second break
  - Repeat 4 times

</td><td>

Day 4: Strength & Balance

- Low lunge to high lunge
  - Move for 60 seconds
  - Repeat on the other side
  - Take a 45 second break
  - Repeat on each side 2 times
- Stork bird
  - Hold for 60 seconds
  - Repeat on the other side
  - Take a 30 second break
  - Repeat on each side 3 times
- Chair pose flow
  - Hold for 45 seconds
  - Take a 30 second break
  - Repeat 3 times
- Warrior III
  - Hold for 45 seconds
  - Repeat on the other side
  - Take a 30 second break
  - Repeat on each side 3 times

</td></tr>
</table>

<table>
<tr><td>

- Half split
  - Hold for 45 seconds
  - Repeat on the other side
  - Take a 30 second break
  - Repeat on each side 3 times
- Reverse warrior flow
  - Move for 30 seconds
  - Repeat on the other side
  - Take a 45 second break
  - Repeat on each side 2 times
- Side bend & reach
  - Move for 30 seconds
  - Repeat on the other side
  - Take a 30 second break
  - Repeat on each side 3 times
- Goddess lifts
  - Move for 60 seconds
  - Take a 45 second break
  - Repeat 3 times

</td><td>

- Seated forward fold
  - Hold for 45 seconds
  - Take a 30 second break
  - Repeat on each side 5 times
- Chair pose flow
  - Move for 60 seconds
  - Take a 30 second break
  - Repeat on each side 4 times
- Palm tree
  - Hold for 60 seconds
  - Repeat on the other side
  - Take a 30 second break
  - Repeat on each side 3 times
- Triangle pose arm rotations
  - Move for 60 seconds
  - Repeat on the other side
  - Take a 30 second break
  - Repeat on each side 5 times
- Standing lunge twist
  - Move for 60 seconds
  - Repeat on the other side
  - Take a 30 second break
  - Repeat on each side 5 times

</td></tr>
</table>

Day 7: Mobility & Strength

- Half goddess steps
  - Move for 45 seconds
  - Take a 30 second break
  - Repeat 3 times
- Goddess revolved ankle touches
  - Move for 30 seconds
  - Take a 45 second break
  - Repeat 3 times
- Low lunge to high lunge
  - Move for 30 seconds
  - Repeat on the other side
  - Take a 30 second break
  - Repeat on each side 3 times
- Chair pose flow
  - Move for 60 seconds
  - Take a 30 second break
  - Repeat 4 times

Day 8: Balance & Stretch

- Tree pose
  - Hold for 60 seconds
  - Repeat on the other side
  - Take a 30 second break
  - Repeat on each side 4 times
- Seated pigeon
  - Hold for 45 seconds
  - Repeat on the other side
  - Take a 30 second break
  - Repeat on each side 3 times
- Overhead shoulder stretch
  - Hold for 30 seconds
  - Take a 30 second break
  - Repeat 3 times
- Palm tree
  - Hold for 60 seconds
  - Repeat on the other side
  - Take a 30 second break
  - Repeat on each side 4 times

Day 9: Cardio & Strength

- Standing lunge twist
  - Move for 60 seconds
  - Repeat on the other side
  - Take a 30 second break
  - Repeat on each side 4 times
- Chair pose flow
  - Move for 60 seconds
  - Take a 30 second break
  - Repeat 5 times
- Goddess side crunches
  - Move for 45 seconds
  - Take a 45 second break
  - Repeat 4 times
- Warrior III crunches
  - Move for 60 seconds
  - Repeat on the other side
  - Take a 30 second break
  - Repeat 5 times

Day 10: Strength & Mobility

- Low lunge to high lunge
  - Move for 30 seconds
  - Repeat on the other side
  - Take a 30 second break
  - Repeat on each side 5 times
- Seated twist
  - Hold for 30 seconds
  - Repeat on the other side
  - Take a 30 second break
  - Repeat on each side 5 times
- Triangle pose arm rotations
  - Move for 30 seconds
  - Repeat on the other side
  - Take a 30 second break
  - Repeat on each side 4 times
- Chair pose flow
  - Move for 45 seconds
  - Take a 30 second break
  - Repeat 5 times

Day 11: Stretch & Balance

- Half split
  - Hold for 60 seconds
  - Repeat on the other side
  - Take a 30 second break
  - Repeat on each side 4 times
- Warrior III
  - Hold for 60 seconds
  - Repeat on the other side
  - Take a 30 second break
  - Repeat on each side 4 times
- Seated forward fold
  - Hold for 60 seconds
  - Take a 30 second break
  - Repeat on each side 4 times
- Stork bird
  - Hold for 60 seconds
  - Repeat on the other side
  - Take a 30 second break
  - Repeat on each side 4 times

Day 12: Mobility & Cardio

- Half goddess steps
  - Move for 60 seconds
  - Take a 30 second break
  - Repeat on each side 2 times
- Reverse warrior flow
  - Move for 30 seconds
  - Repeat on the other side
  - Take a 30 second break
  - Repeat on each side 4 times
- Wide legged forward fold flow
  - Move for 60 seconds
  - Take a 30 second break
  - Repeat on each side 5 times
- Warrior II arm extension
  - Move for 60 seconds
  - Repeat on the other side
  - Take a 30 second break
  - Repeat on each side 5 times

Day 13: Variation

- Half split
  - Hold for 45 seconds
  - Repeat on the other side
  - Take a 30 second break
  - Repeat on each side 5 times
- Low lunge to high lunge
  - Move for 30 seconds
  - Repeat on the other side
  - Take a 30 second break
  - Repeat on each side 3 times
- Tree pose
  - Hold for 60 seconds
  - Repeat on the other side
  - Take a 30 second break
  - Repeat on each side 4 times
- Seated twist
  - Move for 60 seconds
  - Repeat on the other side
  - Take a 30 second break
  - Repeat on each side 3 times
- Side bend & reach
  - Move for 30 seconds
  - Repeat on the other side
  - Take a 30 second break
  - Repeat on each side 2 times

Day 14: Stretch & Strength
- Low lunge backbend
  - Hold for 30 seconds
  - Take a 30 second break
  - Repeat 5 times
- Chair pose flow
  - Move for 60 seconds
  - Take a 30 second break
  - Repeat on each side 5 times
- Seated forward fold
  - Hold for 60 seconds
  - Take a 30 second break
  - Repeat on each side 5 times
- Goddess side crunches
  - Move for 60 seconds
  - Take a 30 second break
  - Repeat 5 times

<table>
<tr><td>

Day 15: Stretch & Strength

</td><td>

Day 16: Balance & Cardio

</td></tr>
</table>

- Low lunge backbend
  - Hold for 45 seconds
  - Release for 30 seconds
  - Repeat 3 times
- Chair pose flow
  - Move for 60 seconds
  - Take a 30 second break
  - Repeat 5 times
- Seated forward fold
  - Hold for 60 seconds
  - Take a 30 second break
  - Repeat 4 times
- Goddess side crunches
  - Move for 45 seconds
  - Take a 45 second break
  - Repeat 3 times

- Palm tree*
  - Hold for 60 seconds
  - Repeat on the other leg
  - Take a 30 second break
  - Repeat each side 3 times
- Wide legged forward fold flow
  - Move for 45 seconds
  - Take a 30 second break
  - Repeat 5 times
- Standing lunge twist
  - Move for 45 seconds
  - Repeat on the other side
  - Take a 30 second break
  - Repeat each side 4 times
- Warrior II arm extension
  - Move for 60 seconds
  - Repeat on the other side
  - Take a 30 second break
  - Repeat each side 3 times

Day 17: Mobility & Stretch

- Triangle pose arm rotations
  - Move for 30 seconds
  - Repeat on the other side
  - Take a 45 second break
  - Repeat each side 2 times
- Seated twist
  - Hold for 30 seconds
  - Repeat on the other side
  - Take a 30 second break
  - Repeat each side 3 times
- Seated pigeon
  - Hold for 60 seconds
  - Repeat on the other side
  - Take a 30 second break
  - Repeat on each side 4 times
- Overhead shoulder stretch
  - Hold for 30 seconds
  - Take a 30 second break
  - Repeat 4 times

Day 18: Strength & Balance

- Low lunge to high lunge
  - Move for 60 seconds
  - Repeat on the other side
  - Take a 45 second break
  - Repeat on each side 2 times
- Stork bird
  - Hold for 60 seconds
  - Repeat on the other side
  - Take a 30 second break
  - Repeat on each side 3 times
- Chair pose flow
  - Hold for 45 seconds
  - Take a 30 second break
  - Repeat 3 times
- Warrior III
  - Hold for 45 seconds
  - Repeat on the other side
  - Take a 30 second break
  - Repeat on each side 3 times

<table>
<tr><td>

Day 19: Stretch & Cardio

- Half split
  - Hold for 45 seconds
  - Repeat on the other side
  - Take a 30 second break
  - Repeat on each side 3 times
- Reverse warrior flow
  - Move for 30 seconds
  - Repeat on the other side
  - Take a 45 second break
  - Repeat on each side 2 times
- Side bend & reach
  - Move for 30 seconds
  - Repeat on the other side
  - Take a 30 second break
  - Repeat on each side 3 times
- Goddess lifts
  - Move for 60 seconds
  - Take a 45 second break
  - Repeat 3 times

</td><td>

Day 20: Mobility & Strength

- Half goddess steps
  - Move for 45 seconds
  - Take a 30 second break
  - Repeat 3 times
- Goddess revolved ankle touches
  - Move for 30 seconds
  - Take a 45 second break
  - Repeat 3 times
- Low lunge to high lunge
  - Move for 30 seconds
  - Repeat on the other side
  - Take a 30 second break
  - Repeat on each side 3 times
- Chair pose flow
  - Move for 60 seconds
  - Take a 30 second break
  - Repeat 4 times

</td></tr>
</table>

Day 21: Balance & Stretch

- Tree pose
  - Hold for 60 seconds
  - Repeat on the other side
  - Take a 30 second break
  - Repeat on each side 4 times
- Seated pigeon
  - Hold for 45 seconds
  - Repeat on the other side
  - Take a 30 second break
  - Repeat on each side 3 times
- Overhead shoulder stretch
  - Hold for 30 seconds
  - Take a 30 second break
  - Repeat 3 times
- Palm tree
  - Hold for 60 seconds
  - Repeat on the other side
  - Take a 30 second break
  - Repeat on each side 4 times

Day 22: Cardio & Strength

- Standing lunge twist
  - Move for 60 seconds
  - Repeat on the other side
  - Take a 30 second break
  - Repeat on each side 4 times
- Chair pose flow
  - Move for 60 seconds
  - Take a 30 second break
  - Repeat 5 times
- Goddess side crunches
  - Move for 45 seconds
  - Take a 45 second break
  - Repeat 4 times
- Warrior III crunches
  - Move for 60 seconds
  - Repeat on the other side
  - Take a 30 second break
  - Repeat 5 times

Day 23: Strength & Mobility

- Low lunge to high lunge
  - Move for 30 seconds
  - Repeat on the other side
  - Take a 30 second break
  - Repeat on each side 5 times
- Seated twist
  - Hold for 30 seconds
  - Repeat on the other side
  - Take a 30 second break
  - Repeat on each side 5 times
- Triangle pose arm rotations
  - Move for 30 seconds
  - Repeat on the other side
  - Take a 30 second break
  - Repeat on each side 4 times
- Chair pose flow
  - Move for 45 seconds
  - Take a 30 second break
  - Repeat 5 times

<table>
<tr><td>

Day 24: Stretch & Balance

- Half split
  - Hold for 60 seconds
  - Repeat on the other side
  - Take a 30 second break
  - Repeat on each side 4 times
- Warrior III
  - Hold for 60 seconds
  - Repeat on the other side
  - Take a 30 second break
  - Repeat on each side 4 times
- Seated forward fold
  - Hold for 60 seconds
  - Take a 30 second break
  - Repeat on each side 4 times
- Stork bird
  - Hold for 60 seconds
  - Repeat on the other side
  - Take a 30 second break
  - Repeat on each side 4 times

</td><td>

Day 25: Mobility & Cardio

- Half goddess steps
  - Move for 60 seconds
  - Take a 30 second break
  - Repeat on each side 2 times
- Reverse warrior flow
  - Move for 30 seconds
  - Repeat on the other side
  - Take a 30 second break
  - Repeat on each side 4 times
- Wide legged forward fold flow
  - Move for 60 seconds
  - Take a 30 second break
  - Repeat on each side 5 times
- Warrior II arm extension
  - Move for 60 seconds
  - Repeat on the other side
  - Take a 30 second break
  - Repeat on each side 5 times

</td></tr>
</table>

Day 26: Stretch & Strength

- Low lunge backbend
  - Hold for 30 seconds
  - Take a 30 second break
  - Repeat 5 times
- Chair pose flow
  - Move for 60 seconds
  - Take a 30 second break
  - Repeat on each side 5 times
- Seated forward fold
  - Hold for 60 seconds
  - Take a 30 second break
  - Repeat on each side 5 times
- Goddess side crunches
  - Move for 60 seconds
  - Take a 30 second break
  - Repeat 5 times

Day 27: Variation

- Overhead shoulder stretch
  - Hold for 60 seconds
  - Take a 45 second break
  - Repeat 3 times
- Goddess side crunches
  - Move for 60 seconds
  - Take a 30 second break
  - Repeat 5 times
- Stork bird
  - Hold for 60 seconds
  - Repeat on the other side
  - Take a 30 second break
  - Repeat on each side 3 times
- Half goddess steps
  - Move for 60 seconds
  - Take a 30 second break
  - Repeat on each side 5 times
- Wide legged forward fold flow
  - Move for 60 seconds
  - Take a 30 second break
  - Repeat on each side 3 times

- Seated pigeon
  - Hold for 60 seconds
  - Repeat on the other side
  - Take a 30 second break
  - Repeat on each side 5 times
- Warrior III crunches
  - Move for 45 seconds
  - Repeat on the other side
  - Take a 30 second break
  - Repeat on each side 4 times
- Warrior III
  - Hold for 45 seconds
  - Repeat on the other side
  - Take a 30 second break
  - Repeat on each side 4 times
- Seated cat/cow
  - Move for 60 seconds
  - Take a 30 second break
  - Repeat 5 times
- Reverse warrior flow
  - Move for 60 seconds
  - Repeat on the other side
  - Take a 30 second break
  - Repeat on each side 5 times

EXERCISE INDEX